Functional Anatomy of Movement

Functional Anatomy
of Movement

An Illustrated Guide to Joint Movement,
Soft Tissue Control, and Myofascial Anatomy

JAMES EARLS

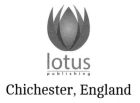

lotus
publishing

Chichester, England

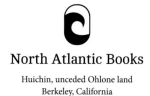

North Atlantic Books

Huichin, unceded Ohlone land
Berkeley, California

First published in 2024 by
Lotus Publishing
Apple Tree Cottage, Inlands Road, Nutbourne, Chichester, PO18 8RJ, and
North Atlantic Books
Huichin, unceded Ohlone land
Berkeley, California

Illustrations Amanda Williams
Text Design Medlar Publishing Solutions Pvt Ltd., India
Cover Design Jasmine Hromjak
Printed and Bound Kultur Sanat Printing House, Turkey

Functional Anatomy of Movement: An Illustrated Guide to Joint Movement, Soft Tissue Control, and Myofascial Anatomy is sponsored and published by North Atlantic Books, an educational nonprofit based on the unceded Ohlone land Huichin (Berkeley, CA), that collaborates with partners to develop cross-cultural perspectives; nurture holistic views of art, science, the humanities, and healing; and seed personal and global transformation by publishing work on the relationship of body, spirit, and nature.

North Atlantic Books' publications are distributed to the US trade and internationally by Penguin Random House Publisher Services. For further information, visit our website at www.northatlanticbooks.com.

Medical Disclaimer: The following information is intended for general information purposes only. Individuals should always see their health-care provider before administering any suggestions made in this book. Any application of the material set forth in the following pages is at the reader's discretion and is their sole responsibility.

British Library Cataloging-in-Publication Data
A CIP record for this book is available from the British Library
ISBN 978 1 913088 38 5 (Lotus Publishing)
ISBN 978 1 62317 841 3 (North Atlantic Books)

Library of Congress Cataloging-in-Publication Data
Names: Earls, James, author. | Williams, Amanda (Illustrator), illustrator.
Title: Functional anatomy of movement : an illustrated guide to joint
    movement, soft tissue control, and myofascial anatomy / James Earls ;
    illustrations Amanda Williams.
Description: Chichester : Lotus Publishing ; Huichin, unceded Ohlone land
    Berkeley, California : North Atlantic Books, 2024. | Includes bibliographical
    references and index.
Identifiers: LCCN 2022057372 (print) | LCCN 2022057373 (ebook) |
    ISBN 9781623178413 (trade paperback) | ISBN 9781623178420 (ebook)
Subjects: LCSH: Musculoskeletal system--Anatomy--Popular works. | Human
    mechanics--Popular works. | Stretching exercises--Popular works.
Classification: LCC QM100 .E23 2024 (print) | LCC QM100 (ebook) |
    DDC 611/.7--dc23/eng/20230510
LC record available at https://lccn.loc.gov/2022057372
LC ebook record available at https://lccn.loc.gov/2022057373

Contents

Acknowledgments

No book appears from a vacuum—each begins with an idea, a suggestion, a hint, and takes off from there. This one began with a request from my long-suffering publisher, Jon Hutchings, who imagined quite a different book would appear in his in-box. Jon, thank you and sorry.

Many people help along the way, mostly my very kind and supportive wife, Liza, who patiently listens to me defend the lack of clarity in my writing and then manages to create order from my chaos.

Others have been drawn in to help along the way—Nicki Mansfield, Owen Lewis, and John Wort, who all saw and read early versions and made helpful contributions along the way; Alex Kolarik, who willingly stood in the right place at the right time and let me take some photographs; and, of course, Amanda Williams, who somehow produces magically clear artwork from my sketchy outlines.

Introduction

I don't know what's the matter with people—they don't learn by understanding, they learn by some other way—by rote or something. Their knowledge is so fragile!

—Richard P. Feynman,
Surely You're Joking, Mr. Feynman!

This is not the book I was asked to write.

My publisher wanted a book of long-chain stretches—a quick and easy project he said—and I agreed. Until I started writing it and looking at the other books already available.

There are already countless books on yoga, Pilates, fascia stretching, easy stretching, sports stretching, relaxation stretching, stretching for menopause, stretching for the elderly, stretching for runners, for swimmers, for cyclists—you name it, there is a title out there for your discipline, life stage, or hobby. Sure, they mostly depict short-chain, isolated-muscle stretches, and a long-chain, whole-body stretch book *could* be different, but would it be helpful? And was that how I wanted to help readers? My problem was

that, to me, books about stretching are all the same. The positions, the instructions, the directions—**all the same**.

This book is not one of those.

I did not want to teach a routine, create a branded sequence of moves with accompanying psychobabble for your enlightenment, nor enter the competition to create the "best 10 stretches" or point out the "15 worst, most dangerous, flawed stretches you should never, ever do again."

Nor did I want to give a recipe book to match symptoms to exercises that are probably just as likely to aggravate as to alleviate. The market has enough of these, not to mention the plethora of social media accounts that insist on giving us more.

This book asks the reader to do some work, but I hope that you are reading it because it is work that you want to do. You have taken the first step toward helping yourself and helping others by buying, borrowing, or stealing it because of what you saw on the front cover, and that fills me with optimism and the belief that you care.

My aim is to help you understand the complexities of movement and to provide some movement ideas to help your clients (and you) by equipping you with a vocabulary of anatomy in motion that will help you to truly see and effectively communicate how the whole body moves. For it is the whole body that moves, never an isolated joint, muscle, or limb.

You care enough to want to understand and to see movement more clearly. The great thing is that both go together—the more I understand, the better I can see. As a psychology student many years ago, I learned that words and vision are connected. If I have a word for something, I can see that thing more clearly. For me, it was the lack of vocabulary for anatomy and movement that stopped me from seeing and understanding movement.

How could I describe movement if I did not know the words with which to do it? For the first 20 years of my practice, there were a lot of words and a lot of very useful conventions that I simply did not know existed—I'd never been taught them in context—and when they were finally first taught to me, I was angry that this could have been overlooked! Sometimes, it seems as though there is a conspiracy to keep this vocabulary a secret—why are the things I have put into this book not taught to therapists and movement teachers from the very beginning? In my angry state it could have been easy for me to conclude that the owners of the trademarked movement disciplines did not want you to know, because if you actually understood movement then you would no longer have to buy their product. But that would have been cynical.

I think the reality is that most authors and schools simply do not know there is a better way to describe anatomy and movement. We all think that we need to follow the rules handed down from teacher to teacher—until one teacher becomes brave enough to change an order, position, or cue.[1]

I hope this book goes some way to ridding us of the lazy educators out there, at least by giving you the facility to explore and develop your own craft, rather than copy and endlessly repeat another's. By working your way through this text, practicing some of the exercises, and developing clarity of the language it provides, you will be able to take control of movement. You will be able to connect movement with anatomy and create your own repertoire.[2]

We will build that skill by first showing the unspoken problems of anatomical position-based anatomy and how it creates limiting prejudices that we are often unaware of. We can then start our journey into movement from the reality of our whole structure and with an appreciation of its interconnectedness and tensegrity-like relationships, which are often interdependent and predictable. The predictability of human movement derives from our shared anatomy, and our anatomy is partially molded through evolution and its drive for efficiency of movement through the interplay among fascia, muscle, and the skeleton.

---

[1] And then goes off to create their own school, with accompanying trademark and branding!

[2] And, if you do trademark it, I want in on it! ;-)

When seeking to understand anything, one of the most powerful questions to ask is "Why?" There are many universal movement strategies, one of which is our tendency to start movements by going backward. We will answer that throughout the text and illustrate many of the reasons why we do it in chapter 3 because, although much has been written in manual and movement therapies about the elastic role of fascia, it has rarely been put in the context of real-world movement patterns. Chapter 3 will lay out how fascial tissue aids optimization of force and velocity outputs—you might recognize some of the graphs—but this text will build the context and put the information into practice through the practical examples given, making it easier for you to transfer the information to application.

One of the major blocks on learning movement is the complexity of how we move—there are almost endless possibilities. Some teachers love to wallow in those convolutions, intricacies, and complications. Rather than disempower you with mystical invocations, I would rather use a vocabulary that empowers you to take control, one that allows you to assess, guide, and predict movement and its reactions through the body. One of the greatest tools for us will be the "planes of movement." I know you may have already seen the planes of movement, and probably moved over them, but, trust me, if you understand what they truly represent and how to use them correctly, they will be your best friend along the journey. The planes of movement will help build the bridge between theory, application, and the vision to see "anatomy in motion."

There is an absolute truth in the complexity of movement, and we can either choose to retain its mystery or acknowledge its universal similarities. Those similarities are inherent within our shared anatomy, but that anatomy also varies from person to person. At different levels, we are all both the same and completely different. Keep this in mind as you venture through the exercises and suggestions. This is not an anatomy book, rather a book that aims to help you understand the differences in movement reactions by seeing the similarities and to provide you with the words to describe them.

Yes, this book asks you to do some work, and it doesn't give all the answers (the publisher wanted a short text!), but if you spend time with it, the dividends are huge.

Functional, not Textbook, Anatomy

Everybody got mixed feelings
About the function and the form.
Everybody got to deviate
From the norm

—Geddy Lee, Alex Lifeson,
Neil Peart, "Vital Signs"

Introduction

My guess is that you are reading this book because, like me, you are searching for new and improved ways to see and understand movement. Perhaps you have suffered through traditional anatomy textbooks and been somewhat confused and disappointed with the world of anatomy because what we read in the books and what we experience in the real world just don't match up. If that is the case you will be glad to know the language, exercises, and images included in this book will guide you to a new, deeper appreciation of vocabulary in ways that will help you see anatomy in movement more clearly.

Time and exposure to numerous approaches to anatomy of movement have helped me

appreciate many reasons why musculoskeletal anatomy is taught in its usual limited and dry manner. Most of the problems are due to the complexity of normal movement, and our anatomy resources cannot cope with the sheer number of variables. Have a look at the variations in figure 1.1. the people are making different movements, in different environments, probably at different speeds and in a range of angles; their feet or pelves have different points of contact with that environment, and they are each using their body with its own unique history of physical training (or lack of), alongside a list of injuries. Talk about complex!

Not only do we each have a physical history but each of us also moves in keeping with our expectations and beliefs around our body and its ability. Those expectations come alongside a wide range of other psychological and emotional considerations that alter the movement strategies we use. Being able to put all those variables and variations into a textbook would not be easy. Thankfully, there are ways in which we can come close to appreciating what is really happening if we understand several principles.

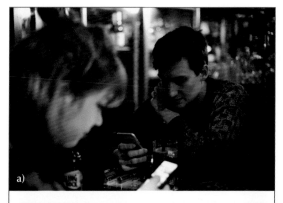

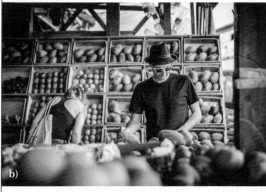

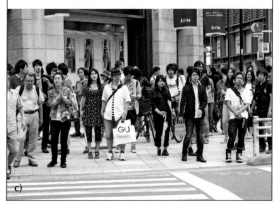

Figure 1.1. Real life requires movement in different positions, at multiple angles, with various speeds. Anatomical position removes many of those variables to give us a simplified story that doesn't fully prepare us for reality.

Most of those principles have been omitted from the anatomy model presented in textbooks but will be included for you here. Importantly, one of the first things we will do

is to break away from the dull and frustrating "anatomical position," with its precise origins and insertions, that gives us those hard-to-remember and limited muscle actions. We will come back to that soon.

Learning Anatomy, the Slow and Hard Way

Textbook anatomy is often taught by people who are older than us, have read more books than us, have been put in positions of authority, and are (too often!) men and, commonly, bearded. They like to use books, large and heavy tomes, with long strange words and terminology that is esoteric and confusing. As students, we are often in awe of these "holders of arcane knowledge," the ones who can speak this strange language with fluency and gravitas. All of this—just like internet conspiracy theories—gives the impression of authority and truth-holding.

We want to be like those professors,[1] but we struggle. Anatomy texts are presented to us as if they carry "The Truth," and we are given the impression that we will be successful if we diligently learn every structure, every attachment, nerve supply, and action. Too often, we become disillusioned before reaching the end of the book.

Well, just as with internet conspiracy theories, you can relax in the knowledge that quite often those professors and the tomes they work from are based on limited understanding of real life.[2] However, many anatomy teachers

---

[1] But with better dress sense and less facial hair.
[2] Please don't mistake my flippancy with disrespect for your wonderful favorite teacher or indeed any other.

do have a much greater vision of anatomy than the books they use, but that vision comes through time with the material. We do not want to take that time—nor is it necessary—and using many of the principles in this text will help you rapidly expand your anatomy. The problem with traditional anatomy is that its standardized ideas about how anatomy should be taught in the first instance come with simplifications, abbreviations, and conventions, which serve us well for the short term but actually create issues as we try to go further into the discipline.

Our anatomy teachers are following a tradition—they are using tools that they are familiar with, tools that have been tried and tested and been found to be …, well, "good enough." Sadly, that "good enough" leaves us with all manner of confusion and frustration. We thought we were getting "The Truth," but in reality it was the "it'll do for now and it's enough to get them through the exam" version.

Reducing the information to the basics, the "just enough to pass the exam" version, instils many unconscious biases and prejudices, which limit and inhibit learning. Unknowingly, traditional anatomy often gets in the way of true understanding.[3]

The Problems with Anatomical Position

The use of anatomical position is probably one of the biggest barriers to understanding functional anatomy. Anatomy books rarely, if ever, tell us that they are presenting us with a model based on several conventions. The conventions used by the books have become so endemic that they are passed down from one author or teacher to the next without question. They are considered an inherent part of the anatomy story and its normal presentation, but each story-telling tradition has a style that prepares the reader for the world they are about to enter. Whether it be the "far away land" of fairy tales or the alcohol-fueled, smoke-heavy scenes of detective noir, the reader is prepared for the world they are about to enter. Anatomy texts don't provide that preparation for us.

One of the problems is the lack of an introductory disclaimer that puts the many assumptions and conventions of the anatomical model into context. By omitting a statement listing those assumptions, the texts are setting us up to experience failure and confusion, as the assumptions are like weeds that grow and get in the way of our path to understanding.

The use of "anatomical position" and its trusty companion, rote memorization of muscles, presents immediate barriers to understanding when we attempt to interpret everyday movement. My eyes were opened to this by the "father of function," Doctor Gary Gray, and his collaborator Professor David Tiberio. I had been teaching anatomy and approaches to anatomy for many years, but it was only when I heard Gray and Tiberio speak of the "Truth of Movement" that I realized how often we try to impose a model of anatomy onto what we see.

I do not want to waste your time with unnecessary introductions to this and that theory. We will get stuck into the nitty

---

[3]The point I am making is that we hold the watered-down story of textbook anatomy too tightly, and our grip on it should be relaxed.

gritty and set the scene for you as quickly as possible by integrating movement suggestions, exploring adaptations, and providing a clear language to describe it all.

Our starting point for the anatomy of movement should not be the textbooks, it should be movement. Movement should inform our interpretation of anatomy, not the other way around. Straight away, there are two major challenges with this new approach—but they exist only because of our previous teachings:

1. As Mr. Rumsfeld famously said, though with less clarity, "We do not know what we do not know." In our case it is the prejudices, the biases, and the unconscious confusions that have been drilled into us through textbook anatomy. Without knowing it, the textbooks have handicapped our ability to grasp the anatomy of movement. This first chapter will expose some of those limitations to help clear the path as we move forward.

2. Because textbook anatomy uses such a small frame of reference, we have not been given the language to describe what we see when people move. Vocabulary and the clarity of language will be an ongoing theme through this text. As parents were so fond of telling their kids, we "need to use our words," and we need to use them correctly. It might seem pedantic, and you may find it a little difficult to grasp initially, but my guarantee to you is, if you practice the language and become fluent in it, you will start to *see* anatomy as it moves.

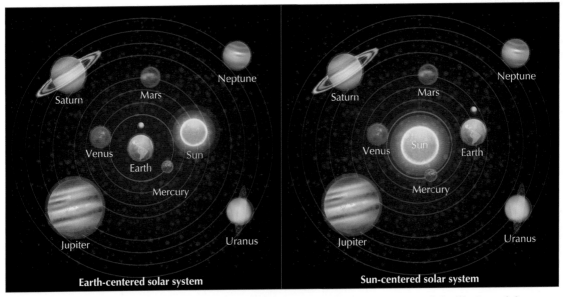

Figure 1.2. Our first observations of the movement of the stars and planets created the illusion of the earth being at the center of the universe. Careful observation of the night sky led Copernicus to develop a better, more accurate model, which held the sun at its center. Copernicus's new model was counter to the teachings of the Church, which believed God had placed humanity at the center of creation. The Catholic Church's strong resistance to the new model is a warning to us that observation, not dogma, should be our starting point for the development of understanding.

Science has a long history of imposing ideas, beliefs, faiths, and models onto reality. For example, reluctance to accept reality over faith hindered the transition from an earth-centered view of the universe to the more accurate sun-centered version (figure 1.2). That new and improved model relied on the principle of parsimony (finding the best-fit explanation for the observations) and underpins scientific development, and we will follow that rule as closely as possible within this short text.

We will fit the anatomy to human movement, not the other way round, which has been the case for too long. It is human movement that should be our starting point for understanding. There are many schools of thought in movement therapies, often with too much dogma and not enough understanding. There are too many trademarked approaches trying to teach us to move in "their" way, with "their" repertoire, and "their" interpretation of anatomy. But there is no "their" anatomy, there is just the anatomy that fits your movement in the context of your body.

So, rather than learning yet another expensive and branded story of movement, let's set off on our ecumenical journey toward the truth of movement and see how anatomy fits to it.

Announcing the Unannounced Rules of Anatomical Position

1. Position

Every listed action in anatomy books begins from anatomical position, but few of us ever find ourselves in that position at any point during the day. Figure 1.1 only gives us a taste of the almost endless variations on body orientation and position from which we must control or create movement. The following chapters will not review every position but will provide you with the tools needed to interpret and predict what is happening in each of them.

We will pay a lot of attention to vocabulary and language skills. The anatomical language for movement is more highly developed than most of us realize. The problem has been the way it has been handed down and diluted over time, with the emphasis being placed on learning location and action rather than the effects of tissues on, and during, movement. Learning that language will take just a little time, and practicing it can be done anytime, anywhere, by simply taking a quiet moment and watching someone as they move.

Each chapter will build your skills of seeing and verbalizing movement. The old saying "Give a man a fish and you feed him for a day, but teach a man to fish and you feed him for a lifetime" is perfect for our approach here. Textbook anatomy gives us fish—lots of them—and because those fish are all in anatomical position, it does not really tell us much about the qualities of fish, their ecology, the ways they like to move, or the best ways to catch them. By the time you have worked through this text, you will be sufficiently prepared to recognize, describe, or design most movements you come across in real life, in the studio, or in clinical practice.

There are reasons why we do not acquire the skills to describe movement during classroom anatomy—there are many more questions to consider than are easy to teach, and the answers are not always clear, exact, or testable. Modern education does not like that level of possible confusion and prefers to deal with absolutes. The anatomy of movement has been simplified by giving us a single position to deal with and has removed most of the other real-world variables.

The ability to name anatomical elements stuck in a single position does not provide flexibility and creativity when you are required to analyze novel movements. Getting below the surface of those words and building fluency in the language of movement and anatomy, however, will give you just that. For example, I was once invited to present at an acrobatic and circus skills symposium. It was one of the scariest and most rewarding conferences I have worked with, and although I had no acrobatic skills or professional exposure to them, I could still put together a coherent analysis of what happens during the many variations of full-body extensions that are required in circus performances.[4]

By the time you finish this text, you will have many new words and a deeper appreciation of how to use the old ones with greater clarity and precision. Having a wider and more accurate vocabulary has been shown time and again to improve one's vision.[5] After working through this text, you will have the skills to describe new and complex movements, even movements that take place in strange and wonderful ways. To benefit from this new vocabulary, however, you must draw on,

_____

[4]Fortunately, the presentation was recorded, and you can judge my success (or lack thereof) for yourself by searching "James Earls Acrobatic Symposium 2015" on YouTube.

[5]To explore the relationship between language and perception I recommend Guy Deutscher's *Through the Language Glass: Why the World Looks Different in Other Languages* (Arrow Books, 2011).

or develop, another strength—you must be prepared to say "I don't know."

Moving away from anatomical position brings increased movement complexity in so many variables that we just cannot always be definitive, and that is OK. The movement patterns and reactions outlined through the text are not absolute but are based on the movement reaction of the normal, average person, who does not exist. However, we must start somewhere, and if we have the idea that there is no "normal movement," then we are left with the assumption that every movement deviation or restriction might be normal. Where does that leave us? It gives us no power, no starting place, no source of questions to investigate for dysfunction or suggestions to help improve.

The pressure to be precise and accurate is part of the illusion delivered within the detail of textbook anatomy. It is almost as if there is a conspiracy to provide us with limited tools to give the impression of exact answers, so that we can perform examinations in ways that can be graded, so that we can apply exact orthopedic tests, so that we can then perform random double-blind controlled tests, so that we can ultimately create standard protocol approaches for each pathology. Thankfully the world is much more interesting and random and far more exciting than that. However, to embrace it we must be content to go to the place of not knowing the final answer.

This text will give you plenty of tools to guide or assess movement that fit for most people, but it cannot give you THE answer for everyone, nor can it provide THE answer for THAT person.[6] But, please, do not put the book away yet! No book can give you all of that, but this book will empower you to start asking better questions—questions that seek answers that will help you and your clients— because we will be looking at all the other variables of movement that were left out of the textbooks.

2. Environment

Our movement environment is probably the biggest movement variable with which we must contend. Part of the excitement and interest of the real world is our constantly changing surroundings. We might be slogging away at the computer desk one day and climbing mountains the next. We make movements while we are sitting, we can swim, and swing from branches, but poor old "anatomy man" only ever gets to float in one place (see below).

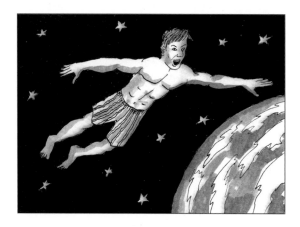

We rarely consider how the anatomical model is somehow floating in space. Let's think about the implications of that for a moment. Its lack of contact with any surface means we only see open-chain movement—for example, the lower limb always moves away from the midline (figure 1.3)—and we are taught anatomy within this tight constraint. As we will see, placing the body in the real world means that the feet are often anchored on the floor as the pelvis moves over the top, and such closed-chain movement changes muscle actions.

The anatomy of movement requires an appreciation of how the environment alters the way forces are dealt with by the body. We will cover many of those variables, but the ability to understand the switch between open- and closed-chain movement and how it affects muscle action is perhaps the biggest breakthrough you can make to help along the way. If these concepts are not familiar to you, don't worry—we will deal with each topic from a range of directions with slightly different vocabulary and images, as it is impossible to explore every possibility up front. We have to present the overriding principles first and then you can practice applying them in your own discipline.

Learning the principles of movement is essential. We cannot take the rote memorization approach used in textbook anatomy. There are an infinite number of ways in which we can change our movement environment. We can have different parts of our body in contact with a surface; the surface could have different properties (think sand versus concrete), it could also be at different angles, or different temperatures, and so on.

---

[6]Look at figure 1.1 again or look at the people around you—anatomical variation is inherent within nature. No two members of any species are identical.

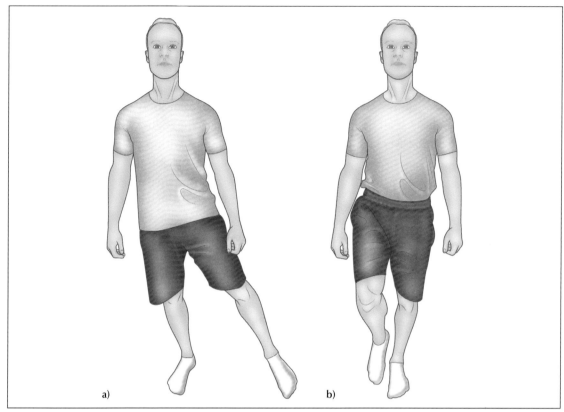

a)　　　　　　　　　　　　　b)

Figure 1.3. (a) Anatomical position and listings of muscle actions generally show only open-chain movement reactions. In open-chain movement the distal attachment is always free to move while the proximal attachment remains fixed. In this case, the left hip abductors are abducting the hip by acting on the femur. (b) But muscles work can work in either direction—their reality is that they can pull on either bone they are attached to and they can also move their proximal attachment. By pulling downward on the iliac crest, the left hip abductors are also creating abduction at the left hip joint. The effect of that pull will depend on intention and environment. Quite often, the distal bone is fixed (closing the chain) and the proximal bone can be moved, stabilized, or controlled as it moves away. We will keep circling back to further clarify these issues as we progress through the text.

3. The Missing Forces

Somehow "anatomy man" lives in a world with no gravity, ground reaction force, friction, or momentum present. To "see" anatomy in action, we must understand the effect each force has on the body. We will address each of them through the text, but don't panic—there will be very few graphs and even fewer equations, I promise. This is not a standard biomechanics text. My intention is to develop the language and therefore the vision to "*see*" anatomy, not to pass college tests.

Jargon, unnecessarily complicated equations, and questionable science have all hindered our understanding of normal, real-life movement. The aim here is to give you a working appreciation to see how the forces interact to change how our tissue reacts. The reality is that most of us don't really care or need to know how to measure the forces acting on and through the body, we just want to understand how it moves (or doesn't), and so we can leave the kinetic side of biomechanics to those who are inclined that way.

Figure 1.3 shows the different actions of the hip abductors during open- and closed-chain movements, but it also presents the effects of gravity, momentum, and ground reaction forces. We will explore the forces of gravity, ground reaction force, and momentum, but it is worth defining them briefly here first.

We will consider **gravity** to be constant in both direction and the amount of force it applies to the body. Although more people might be popping into space thanks to Mr. Bezos very few of us are likely to be experiencing zero gravity anytime soon. Gravity does change slightly with altitude but not to such a degree that it really affects our movement, and if you are that high, the lack of oxygen will be more of a concern than how your "glutes" might be working.

While gravity might be constant, **ground reaction force** is highly variable and, just to confuse us a little, it is not always a *ground* reaction force. Reaction forces result from any interaction with a surface, but the most discussed reaction force is the one we feel from the ground with every step. If you are sitting to read this text, your chair or sofa is supporting you by providing a reaction force. Move slightly in the chair and you can sense the change in pressure under your pelvis as the angle of that pressure alters accordingly.

The degree of pressure also changes according to the material properties of the surface. If you are sitting on a relatively hard chair, you will feel more pressure compared with the soft and cushioning sofa. Your body weight has not changed during the walk between one piece of furniture and the next, it is the sofa's ability to "cushion" the pressure by distributing it through its softer materials that gives the impression of less pressure.

Different ground surfaces will do the same thing—this is why running on sand is harder work than running on a road (because the softer/more dispersible surface absorbs a larger percentage of the impact force), and why running on a road can be more jarring to our system (because the harder surface absorbs less of the impact force, which is why we try to change the environment for our feet and purchase "cushioning" trainers).

Surfaces also provide various degrees of friction. Consider the difference between walking along a path on a summer's day and doing so after a winter's frost (figure 1.4). It may be the same path, the same incline, and even a similar reaction force, but your gait will not be the same. Your stride is likely to shorten if you sense a danger of slipping on ice as you instinctively want to increase the angle at which your foot contacts the ground, meaning your soft tissues have to adjust to the new rhythm and pace as you reduce your speed. Reduced speed will affect how your muscles work, as forces created through momentum can be used to load energy into elastic tissues and be recycled to reduce muscle work.

Momentum is a major factor in real-life movement. Muscle-action-based anatomy assumes it is muscles that create the force to move us, but that is not always the case. Think about what happens after you throw a

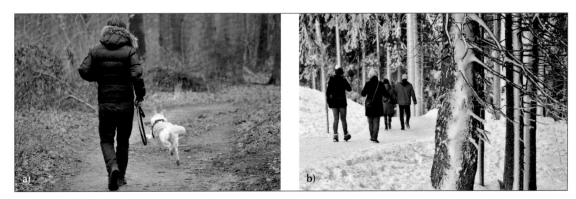

Figure 1.4. (a) A relaxed walk allows us to optimize the relationship of forces through the body and balances the forces of gravity, ground reaction force, momentum, and friction for efficiency. (b) We instinctively shorten our stride when walking on icy surfaces. A shorter step length increases the angle between the ground and the foot and reduces the chances of slipping on the low-friction ice. The chances of slipping are lessened because the ground reaction force and gravity are brought closer to each other.

ball—your body responds to the momentum of your arm, and your spine and hips will probably flex, but not necessarily because of contractions from the flexor muscles. We will see many examples of how, because it is completely connected, the body transfers movement through itself—movement in one body part should create movement elsewhere.

4. Joint-Specific Movement

Anatomical-position anatomy assumes only the joints crossed by the muscle tissue are the ones affected by the muscle's contraction. This is a strong prejudice and is even embedded in how we name many muscles. Using their anatomical-model "actions," we name muscles directly according to their actions (e.g., flexor hallucis longus and adductor brevis), and we group muscles together according to their common actions (e.g., the abductors, the plantar flexors). The language is so ingrained that when we hear the "abductors" being

talked about, we know it is the hips under discussion. As we will see, this common language can be very useful as a shorthand—it allows us to know exactly where we are, and which tissues are being addressed—but it harbors unseen prejudices that limit our thinking. Do the "abductors" only abduct? No, they also control adduction and can produce and control medial and lateral rotation, as well as flexion and extension of the hip, so why do we insist on lumping them together, and thereby limiting them, as "abductors?"

As every muscle will affect joints and tissues beyond its defined span of "origin and insertion," we will build toward a full-body, interactive, and interrelated vision and see how changes in tone of a muscle can ripple outward beyond its attachment sites. For example, stand up and balance on your right leg, but let your hip drop (figure 1.5), and then use your hip abductors to bring your pelvis back to horizontal again.

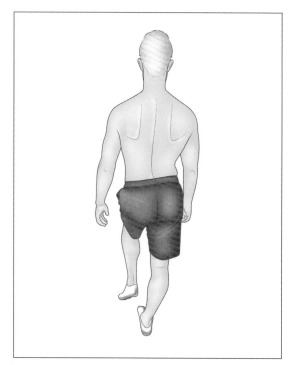

Figure 1.5. Start by maintaining the pelvis in the horizontal plane and then slowly let it drop on the left, and then bring it back to horizontal. This simple exercise reveals some of the limitations of anatomical-position-based anatomy, which generally lists only concentric open-chain actions. In this case, the hip abductors on the right are working isometrically (no change in length) to stabilize the pelvis, then eccentrically to allow the proximal bone (the ilium) to move away from the femur, and finally concentrically to return the pelvis to horizontal. We will explore this further in figure 1.7.

Of course, other muscles were involved, and we need to appreciate how other muscles play supporting roles during movement, as no muscle—nor group of muscles—works independently.

For example, in the exercise in figure 1.5 our need to stay relatively aligned to gravity (i.e., to remain upright) requires the spine to bend

as the pelvis tilts away. The bend of the spine helps the head stay in place, but then try keeping your head, spine, and pelvis neutral to one another as the right hip adducts to see what would happen—it can't be done without falling over (see figure 1.7). Although this simple movement is something we do with every step, anatomical position and its associated language makes it confusing because of its failure to appreciate the influence of gravity and the interconnectedness of the body.

5. Muscle Action—Not Function

Following on from the reality of the interrelated joint action is its consequence for the coordinated reaction through many groups of muscles that must act in concert with one another to create, control, or prevent movement. In contrast to the reality of the body's interconnectedness, anatomical position allows only the distal bone to move in response to a muscle contraction, but in the real world that is rarely the case. It is only when confined by exercise equipment, or the instructions of certain disciplines such as Pilates or yoga, or by other environmental factors, that movement is limited to one or two joints. That is not to say that any of those restrictions are necessarily bad things—they add precision and control to a discipline, focusing strength or motor control into specific areas.

Anatomical-position-based anatomy has given us the impression that we can use isolated muscle actions to create exercises. The ability to focus strength and control into precise areas for a client can be an extremely useful tool for any therapist—movement or manual— but it has generally been done in a shotgun manner. By "shotgun," I mean that anatomical-position-based understanding has bred the idea of general toning and control without the appreciation of *why* the exercises are being done—we just know that giving a range of exercises will probably hit the target, just as sending a spray of pellets from the barrel of a gun is likely to hit something.

There are many books to show what curls, squats, and lunges do for your "glutes," or how various asanas or other repertoires can "improve your core." Few books exist to show how any of that relates to real-life movement and *why* you might want to use precise exercises for the client in front of you at that time. An aim of this book is to give you the tools to provide a truly holistic, individual program to match the needs of your client in that moment. However, this book does not aim to give you prescriptions. It is not embedded within any one philosophy, dogma, or aesthetic, as I believe we must match the intervention to the energy of the client.[7]

My favorite example of textbook thinking is the "weak glutes" epidemic highlighted by many social media posts over the last decade.[8] With dubious evidence, weak glutes have been blamed for weak feet, weak knees, and weak sacroiliac joints. One common exercise to rebuild strength in those poor weak glutes is the clam (figure 1.6), an exercise that has also launched many social media posts with long

comment threads, as it excites many keyboard warriors into paroxysms owing to its lack of *Functional* authenticity.[9]

Although the clam exercise might not replicate the most common function of the glutes, it can still be very useful because it provides an easy-to-perform, do-it-anywhere (within reason and decency!) exercise. The clam is recognized by most people, and the majority can achieve some degree of mastery and gain noticeable benefits quickly. For those reasons, the clam may be *the* ideal exercise in matching some clients' energy. Not every client wants to be lunging in the middle of a room swinging their arms around.

I would argue that it is not the exercise, nor the environment, that makes an exercise *functional*; rather, it is my understanding of how that exercise relates to everyday movement and might assist my client in rebuilding trust to perform it.

What Is Functional Exercise?

You can know the name of that bird in all the languages of the world, but when you're finished, you'll know absolutely nothing whatever about the bird.... So, let's look at the bird and see what it's doing—that's what counts.

—**Richard P. Feynman,**
What Do You Care What Other People Think?

---

[7] I use "energy" in its widest and loosest sense—you can interpret it as you see fit according to your own belief system or therapeutic approach. To me, it seems an appropriate word to cover many of the biopsychosocial variables that should all be considered when working with a client and, as such, serves as a catch-all term.

[8] Where would we be without those online gurus?

[9] Yes, Functional with a capital "F" because for many of those keyboard warriors, replication of function is **everything** and the clam just does not fit that bill.

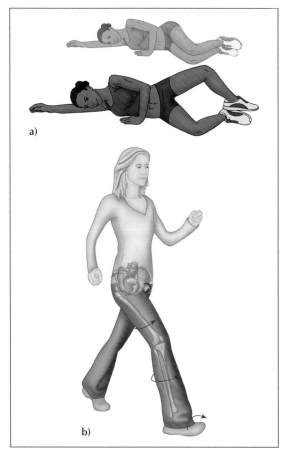

a)

b)

Figure 1.6. (a) "Weak glutes" and "nonfiring glutes" have been blamed for numerous pathologies, and clients have often been prescribed the clam exercise as part of their rehabilitation. While there are many benefits to the clam exercise, one of the negative side effects of its prescription is that it reinforces the limitations of anatomical position. During the clam exercise, the femur moves away from the pelvis, an abduction of the hip with some lateral rotation, almost the exact description of the action of gluteus maximus. (b) Contrast the exercise with the function of gluteus maximus during gait. Following heel strike, the glutes must decelerate hip adduction, flexion, and medial rotation. In this case, gluteus maximus does not perform its "actions"—rather than accelerate, or enable, hip abduction or lateral rotation, it must act functionally to decelerate the opposite movements.

As the famous physicist Richard Feynman points out in the quote above, knowing the names of anatomical bits does not provide an understanding of what they do. We need to look beyond the individual elements and see them in context. This book aims to be ecumenical in its approach to movement—there are many styles, disciplines, schools of thought, and anatomical variations that could be covered when discussing how humans move. I do not aim to analyze, correct, or challenge any of them, as they all have a place and each can help people live happier, healthier lives. There is a movement style out there to gel with each therapist, and, in turn, each therapist will find the clients who connect with that style. My hope is that the application of our interventions will be enhanced if we can understand the rationales behind them.

Rather than attacking the clam exercise, let's understand what it does and what it does not do. If we want to claim it is not *functional*, then we should understand what "normal" movement is (if we consider normal, everyday movement to be the defining character of *functional*). So, it is at this point that we should define the difference between the anatomy of functional, everyday movement and *functional movement and exercise.*

They have much in common: three-dimensionality of movement, an appreciation of gravity, ground reaction forces, and momentum, along with the multidirectionality of muscle forces. However, *functional exercise* can be applied without any understanding or deep appreciation of everyday anatomy or how the body moves when it is walking, running, reaching for the plates in the top cupboard, or sweeping the floor. Exercises can be created to mimic all of those actions, to build up strength and coordination, and those can be *functional*, but my belief is that any exercise only really becomes functional when the therapist *understands* how it helps build toward greater success for that client.

For that reason, I contend that a clam (or any other "isolated" exercise) can be just as functional as any funky arm waving performed in the middle of the room. What defines the functionality of an exercise is not its novelty, its three-dimensionality, the new-fangled piece of equipment similar to something our ancestors might have used, or the fact that one does it barefoot in a freezing stream—the functionality of an exercise comes down to the fact that I have a clear goal for my client and that I have suggested a specific exercise to help their safe and successful progression toward better, safer, less painful movement.

Rather than attack or undermine any exercise, we can take a step back and just ask ourselves what is going on during the exercise and what its qualities and characteristics are that we could use to help with a client.[10] To return to the clam example above, the *Functional* fans claim it doesn't replicate the real action of the glutes, and that might be true. But do we all understand what the real actions are? Do we know what direction and when each of the glutes will "fire" and by how much? And do we know which other muscles, joints,

and tissues will be adapting to facilitate the movement?

To answer each of those questions in turn for every possible movement would require a much larger and much less entertaining book. Human movement is extremely variable, and the firing of the glutes will depend on whether one is walking uphill, downhill, along a flat road, getting up from a chair, or … add any of your own possibilities. This book does not aim to give you those answers but to provide you with the vocabulary and the skills to answer them for yourself regardless of the novelty of any midstream, arm-waving, barefoot, javelin-throwing squat variation you might be asked to analyze.

Gaining that vocabulary will require breaking down some of the many unconscious prejudices that were quietly instilled during the rote learning of anatomical-position-based anatomy. So much time was spent on the naming and listing of muscles according to the effect they had on the joints they crossed that we neglected to see how the rest of the body reacts during movement. For example, as alluded to above, the hip abductors used in the clam exercise match the textbook action (more or less), but the abductors can control *ad*duction, and they have to do so with every step we take—in a controlled manner—and that creates a whole new set of things for us to consider.

If we are standing, walking, or running and we allow one hip to adduct, what happens to our head? Do we let our head follow the tilt of the pelvis? Perhaps in some cases, but usually not. To prevent our eyes ticktocking back and forth

---

[10]Because, after all, walking backward is a good functional and Functional exercise!

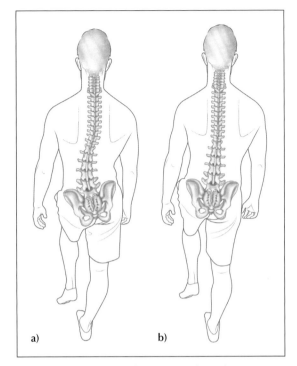

a)

b)

Figure 1.7. (a) Repeat the exercise from figure 1.5 by standing on your right leg and allow your pelvis to drop down to the left. Feel how your rib cage remains relatively vertical, indicating that the spine must have side bent to reduce the tilt between your pelvis and thorax. (b) Now, focus on your right abductors and use them to draw your pelvis back to horizontal. As the pelvis comes back to level, the spine straightens. The straightening of the spine is a reaction to the contraction of your hip abductors—that is, the hip abductors influence the movement and the position of the spine, not just the pelvis and the femur.

as we walk, we allow the spine to side bend as the hips adduct and abduct, and so there are numerous knock-on effects through the body. Try the exploration shown in figure 1.7 to start building a greater sense of these interrelationships.

Important Experiential Note

Awareness of why you might not feel the same reaction through your body as I have described when you work through some of the exercises is vital to grasping the teachings in this text. It can be useful to work through many of the movements with a study partner or in a classroom situation, as you might not be able to see or feel the reasons why, for example, your left foot did not pronate, or your spine didn't react the way you imagined.

Having more eyes and more brainpower applied to the problem will accelerate your learning. It will help you practice the vocabulary and expand your vision as you can explore each other's reaction in each exercise.

Contracting Muscles and Opening Minds

One of the things you might have noticed in the exercise in figure 1.7 is that we just used the "abductors" in two different directions. First, they worked to decelerate the *ad*duction of the right hip, and then they were used to lift the hip (and spine!) back to neutral. However, it is only the latter "action," the *ab*duction (and only that hip movement), that is normally listed in the textbooks.

Only the concentric, shortening action of the muscle is traditionally listed, but to understand the functions of the abductors we had to include its eccentric (the controlled lengthening into hip adduction as the iliac crest moves away from the femur) and isometric abilities (holding the pelvis level), as well as the concentric (the return to a horizontal pelvis). Although the ability to list concentric actions is highly regarded in most examinations, to start "seeing" movement one must be free from the blinkers of assuming movement is created by concentric actions. This unblinkered vision becomes especially useful when we add other forces into the mix, because real-world movement occurs through constant adjustments in the tone of muscles as their contractile fibers react to a complex blend of momentum, gravity, and ground reaction force (figure 1.8).

Many people have found it useful to reconsider muscles as stiffness adjusters within the myofascial system. Muscles will constantly change their tone to match your current movement needs. A little more tone to prevent your collapse under the influence of gravity and ground reaction forces, a bit less tone to allow the front of the hip to open as the

momentum of the other leg swings through, or a lot more "glute" tone to help push you up the hill. Simply, muscles monitor the relationships between bones, and they allow, prevent, or create movement, depending on our needs and our abilities.

As we saw in the exercise in figure 1.7, a muscle's tone not only controls the relationship between the bones it attaches to, it also affects the rest of the body. Widening our vision of how muscles can influence beyond their traditionally accepted borders reveals the fallibility of another textbook tradition— "origin" and "insertion."

The idea of origins and insertions is gradually becoming less popular and being replaced by the more honest proximal and distal attachment, but even this new terminology can inhibit our appreciation of the wider, real-life influence of a muscle. But using proximal and distal attachments to describe a muscle's position at least gives us the ability to remove the open-chain prejudice inherent within textbook listings of actions.

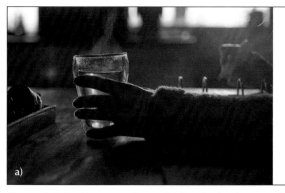 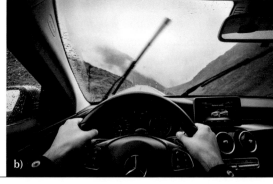

Figure 1.8. During everyday activities the body naturally swaps back and forth between open- and closed-chain movement. The most common pattern is for the upper limbs to move in open chain as we reach for our glasses, cups of coffee, or the steering wheel, while our lower body carries out closed-chain actions as the feet stay in contact with the floor, or the pelvis is perched on a seat.

Although few of us are told about it, the origin and insertion tradition was based on the assumption of the insertion being the attachment that moved toward the origin, but, once again, that was based on the fantasy world of anatomical position. Anatomical position assumes every movement is internally created by the muscle under investigation and that the distal bone is free to move, but, as we have already seen, this is not always the case. In the real world, we must cope with closed-chain movement, where bits of us might be stuck on the ground, in a chair, or grasping an overhead bar. These fixations of distal limbs, our back, or our pelvis by elements within the environment will reverse the actions and allow the muscle to control the proximal rather than the distal bone.

Vocabulary Builder—Defining Movement

Although it might seem like an obvious thing to point out, it is important that we clarify the language of position and movement because sometimes we can get a little muddled.

Let's take the example from the pelvis-dropping exercise above (see figure 1.7) when we abducted and adducted the right hip joint. We were happy to describe the hip as neutral when standing quietly with both feet on the floor, and hopefully you managed to keep the right hip close enough to neutral when you lifted your left foot. You might have deviated and wiggled a little but I expect you were happy enough and within the neutral range—that you did not expect yourself to stay

in anatomical neutral, and you gave yourself some leeway.

Then we let the pelvis drop on the left and the right hip adducted before we brought it back up to neutral. So, we started close to neutral, the hip adducted into an adducted position and then came back to neutral by *ab*ducting the right hip joint, but yet the hip did not go into abduction, it returned to neutral. This is where many people get tied up as we use similar words to describe both the position of joints and movement at the joints.

When we use the suffix "-ion" with a joint descriptor it usually means the joint is in that position—the joint may be in, or going into, flex*ion*, extens*ion*, abduc*tion*, medial rota*tion*, and so on.

When we use the suffix "-ing," it means only that the joint is moving in that direction—it does not tell us how far the joint moves, where it started from, or where the movement ends. For example, if I say "my hip is flex*ing*," we know only the direction in which it is moving. I have not said whether it is going into flex*ion* or not. I might have started flexing my hip from an extended position and brought it back to neutral.

The suffix "-ed" is tense specific. If I say "my hip is flex*ed*," it usually means that it is flexed relative to the neutral of anatomical position. But I can also use "flex*ed*" to describe the movement that took place, as in "I *flexed* my hip to bring it back to neutral again." From this sentence, I must assume that the hip was extended before I started the movement.

If that last sentence didn't quite make sense, please read it again. Maybe reread the description of the hip exercise in figure 1.7—once the right hip was *ad*ducted, we then *ab*ducted it back to neutral again. We could also say that the hip went into *ad*duction and then came back to neutral using *ab*duction. For most of us these sentences make sense in context, and it is only when someone tries to explain how the words can or should be used that they become confusing. So, if you were happy with the descriptors before we started, then be reassured that this section is here for you anytime you need to pass the confusion on.

Don't Panic—All Was Not Wasted

At this stage you could be forgiven for thinking that anatomical position serves no purpose and should be thrown out altogether, but there was a reason why the concept developed. To communicate and to measure anything we need some form of standard measurement, a starting point, a reference, or a universally agreed convention. Anatomical position gives us that point of reference. It is the neutral position from which we can describe changes, and having an agreed-upon starting point makes communication of ideas much easier and can help us avoid expensive mistakes.

Confusion and miscommunications are rife without a commonly agreed reference point and language. For example, the $125 million Mars Climate Orbiter spacecraft launched by NASA in 1999 was destroyed because a supplier used imperial measurements for its calculations, while NASA used the scientific standard metric. As the craft drifted off course during its orbit, there was confusion in Houston because no matter how many corrections were made through its boosters, the spacecraft could not come back to the correct flight path.

Although NASA might have accepted the metric units used by the rest of the world, much of the rest of the US still retains the older (and more confusing) "English" or "imperial" units. The metric system was originally based on interrelated measurements of meters, liters, and kilograms. Although the definitions have been refined and improved on as the tools of science evolve, it was the French who first adopted something like the modern metric system after the Revolution of 1789–99, in an effort to refine the unwieldy earlier weights and measurement system that had developed through the country. Up to that point, each town and trade could have its own system, and royalty could change the standards on a whim. The lack of a countrywide measurement caused all kinds of problems, especially the swindling of the less educated populace.

In search of *égalité* and to improve *fraternité*, French scientists agreed to define a meter as one ten-millionth of the distance from the equator to the North Pole (figure 1.9). From this standard, proposed in 1793, the French Academy of Sciences then defined the liter as a cubic decimeter of water. A standard measure of weight was then created as a liter of water was deemed to weigh a kilogramme (also spelled "kilogram" and commonly shortened to "kilo").

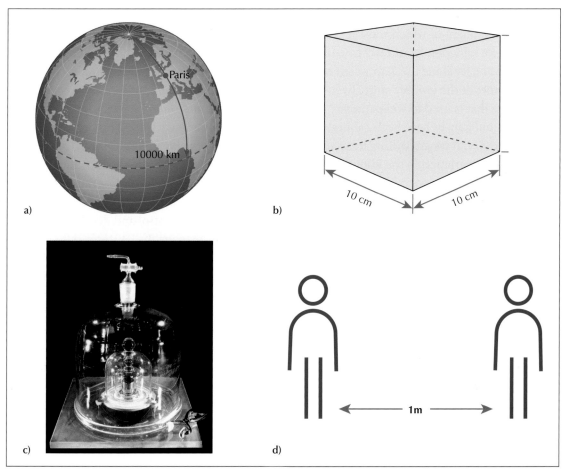

Figure 1.9. Quantifying and communicating change requires measurement, and measurement requires the establishment of a standard from which change can be quantified. Length was standardized first: the meter was defined as one ten-millionth of the distance from the equator to the North Pole (a). As the system is decimal, the meter can then be divided into hundredths (centimeters) and tenths (decimeters). Then volume (b): the liter was defined as a cubic decimeter (10 × 10 × 10 cm). Finally, weight: the kilogram (c) was defined as the weight of a liter of water.

Although further improvements have enhanced the accuracy of these measurements, the intention was to remove the variability of the previous system, which used body-based units such as the *inch* (the width of an average man's thumb across the nail) and *foot* (strangely enough, the length of the average foot).

Although some mourn the change away from body-based reference points, the metric system provided "earth-centered" references and moved away from the egocentricity of using the human body, which had led to inconsistency and, like most "human-centered" activities, was prone to corruption and misinterpretation.

It is unlikely that any of us will even see Le Grand K (the weight of which was the official definition of a kilogram from 1889 to 2019; see figure 1.9c), let alone use it to weigh our bag of potatoes at the grocery store. Even the measure that is used to weigh those groceries is unlikely to have been calibrated by Le Grand K, but we are willing to accept some degree of variation in the kilogram weights we use.

Anatomical position is our base, it is our "Le Grand K" for description of movement and relationships through the body. However, unlike the perfect kilo, anatomical position should be held quite loosely when dealing with clients. Anatomical neutral has sometimes been mistaken for ideal or balanced posture, but that ideal should be put into the context of the individual, who varies and differs from every other individual. The idea of neutral, perfect posture gives us a baseline from which we can ask ourselves if something has caused us or our client to change in a way that alters our movement potential.

Rather than thinking of anatomical position as a goal, or the ideal, see it rather as an agreed-upon standard from which we can describe and measure anything that varies from that position. Anatomical position gives us an anchor for the descriptive language of movement. It is the reference point for the words we use. Without a starting position, we would be anchor-less and have no frame of reference from which we could name movements as they are happening, but we will benefit from some exploration of the nuances.

To understand functional anatomy, we must appreciate:

1. Movement can start from any feasible position (as seen in figure 1.1).
2. The environment will have a significant influence on what can or cannot move (have a look at *the phone-user in figure 1.1a, the table and chair are inhibiting movement in the lower body, but that is not true for the guy choosing his fruit in figure 1.1b*).
3. Muscles work within a rich context of forces acting on the body—not only do muscles help produce momentum, they also work to control and decelerate it. Muscles manage the constant influence of gravity and variable ground reaction forces (if these are less familiar to you, do not panic—we will put them into context for you later).
4. Real-life movement recruits multiple joints. It is only during orthopedic assessments when using specialized exercise equipment that we isolate a single joint.
5. Muscles can create reactions beyond their borders, and they work in groups and interact with their surrounding and supporting fascial tissues and bones.
6. Muscle fibers work to create, control, and decelerate movement. We have to consider their eccentric and isometric abilities as well as their concentric actions.

The principles for functional movement include:

1. **Multiple positioning options**
2. **Environmental influences**
3. The presence of **gravity**, **reaction forces**, **momentum**, and **friction**
4. **Multijoint reactions** to movement

5. **That muscles are influenced by and influence movement beyond their borders**
6. **That muscles function in open- and closed-chain actions**, and can respond to movement by lengthening, shortening, or maintaining their length (eccentric, concentric, or isometric contractions, respectively).

We will explore and expand on each of the principles of functional movement as we progress through the text and build a wider vocabulary. That vocabulary will help us understand how each of the principles outlined above assists our vision of movement.

Reflection Questions

1. What were your frustrations when first learning anatomy?
2. What areas do you struggle with?
3. What are your aims for this book—what would you like to achieve from it? Stating these now will help you identify and focus on the important areas for you.
4. How would you define "functional movement"?
5. What are the important differences between saying a joint is *flexed* and saying that it is *flexing*?

Notes

This book, especially the clarification of our vocabulary, owes a lot to what I learned during a functional movement training with Doctor Gary Gray and Professor David Tiberio of the Gray Institute. I can thoroughly recommend their GIFT mentorship program, which I completed in 2012. The GIFT program is expensive, but I have never met anyone who has regretted the investment.

Copernicus and the move to a geocentric universe: In between reading books on anatomy and evolution I enjoy the occasional sidetrack into the history of science. I wish more people also did this as I have learned much from it, not just from knowing where and why insights came about but also from the humility it teaches. That humility is born from the well-established fact that what is considered fact today is probably on its way to being fiction tomorrow. Fewer on-line debates would be necessary if we all understood that we should hold our current "facts" loosely.

The story of the Mars Climate Orbiter is readily available on many websites, but the ever-reliable Wikipedia page can be found here—https://en.wikipedia.org/wiki/Mars_Climate_Orbiter.

American readers may be less familiar with the metric system compared with the everyday "English units" (known as Imperial units elsewhere). Once again, Wikipedia may prove a useful initial resource for further information.

Why Do We Move the Way We Do?

It turns out that all life is interconnected with all other life.

—**Richard P. Feynman,** *The Meaning of It All: Thoughts of a Citizen Scientist*

Introduction

Human movement is complex. As we have seen in chapter 1, anatomy teachers have tried to simplify it with certain rules and conventions to make it more understandable. However, these simplifications sometimes get in the way, limiting our perception and creating as much confusion as clarification. In chapter 1 we reviewed the purpose of some of the conventions and rules. In this chapter we will observe some of the ways humans move and put that in context by looking into the past and comparing the movement of modern humans with that of our ancestors and ape relatives.

Just as one might do when walking a trail, taking a few steps back helps us see where we have come from. By looking back, we can review the context of our journey so far and understand how we got here. We also get the opportunity to see the same features from a different viewpoint, one that might give greater appreciation and insight into the landscape in which we find ourselves.

The complex range of human movement strategies has developed because of our history. Every animal has preferred methods of locomotion, but the human body appears capable of a much wider range of options than most other species—we can walk, run, climb, and swim. However, we don't excel at much—there are smoother swimmers, faster runners, and more adept climbers. Although we may excel at efficient distance walking and running, I think it is fair to say that our specialism is probably the variety of movement options open to us.

How the Need to Survive Has Shaped Us

Such a wide range of movement possibilities might cause problems for describing human motion unless we take several steps back and appreciate some of the basic principles of our biology. For example, we all know that humans have spines and—along with 70,000 other species—belong to a group of animals known as *vertebrates*. Birds, amphibians, reptiles, and mammals are all vertebrates, and, although we all have different methods of moving around, we share a very similar skeleton because we have a shared ancestry (figure 2.1).

Although we might be awed by the range of swimmers, fliers, and runners in the vertebrate camp, they account for only about 5% of animal species. The other 95% of species do not have spines but have diverse body plans ranging from the hard exoskeletons of beetles to the soft segmented bodies of worms. As Darwin informed us, each species has evolved within its ecology to find a successful balance between its energy needs, its ability to procreate, and its skill in avoiding being eaten before it can produce its progeny.

Although vertebrates make up only 5% of the world's animal population, they are the species we are most familiar with, a fact that partly comes down to size. One of the most noticeable differences between vertebrates and invertebrates is volume (size), and it is the vertebrate's internal skeleton that provides a framework dense enough for the animal to grow larger, wander on land, and work against gravity.

Having dense material inside our human body provides some stability to it and reduces the amount of squeezing that would be necessary to keep us upright if we were made up of wormlike soft-tissue segments. There are some large invertebrates—like the giant octopus, which can grow to a span of over 14 feet (4.3 meters), but it can grow to that volume only because of the support given by the ocean it swims in. An octopus—or any of the cephalopod family—is fascinating to watch. Take a moment to contrast the movement potentials between octopus and human bodies. If you haven't already, watch some YouTube videos of octopuses escaping from predators, solving puzzles, and manipulating their environment. Their ability to squeeze through crevices and morph themselves to blend into their surroundings is partly due to having no skeleton.

Cephalopods like the octopus have no bone or cartilage, just a beak made of chitin for chewing, and their limbs are purely muscular hydrostats. Although you might not recognize the term, we are all familiar with the trunk of an elephant. Like octopus limbs, the trunk works along the principles of a muscular hydrostat—a complex system of muscle fibers arranged in alternating directions on different layers, with "interstitial" fluid between the many surfaces to enable differential movement of each layer. This layered system forms a mobile "bag" that gains stability by compressing its fluid contents. That might sound unusual, and you might not thank me for the image, but we all possess the same arrangement in our mouths.

Variability of movement is an essential part of food processing. We move food around our mouths from one area to another to ensure adequate chewing. Even swallowing our food and ensuring it goes down the right tube—the esophagus and not the trachea—requires a highly mobile tongue. The tongue's potential for movement is underrated by most of us.

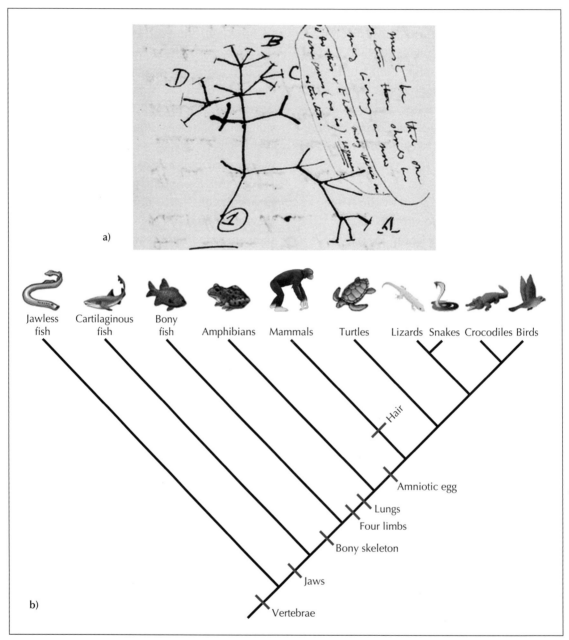

Figure 2.1. (a) Darwin first sketched his idea of the treelike branching arrangement of the evolution of life in 1837. The treelike image should not be interpreted as indicative of a progression or advancement—rather, it is simply a convenient form to represent the relationships between organisms. (b) Groups of animals evolved from earlier animal forms; all were formed by adaptation of the DNA of those that came before them. We think of birds, reptiles, and mammals as being quite different, but, because they all belong to the vertebrate group, they share many skeletal similarities despite differing in whether they have, for instance, a jaw, a bony rather than cartilaginous skeleton, or lungs.

Only speech therapists and voice coaches tend to take a deep interest in this wonderful tool—and it is wonderful because its directional movement is almost limitless.

Contrast your tongue's movement around your mouth with the potential motion between your humerus and ulna. The density of the upper limb bones and the arrangement at the elbow joint create limits that do not exist for the tongue.

Read that short paragraph again, but read it aloud—or silently if you prefer, but let your mouth move with the words. Be aware of the harmonious symphony of coordinated movement between your tongue and your lips—can you imagine trying to speak with a jointed tongue or bony lips? It might be disconcerting to think that we have something resembling a squid tentacle in our mouth but the tongue's malleability—its shape-shifting form—is an essential part of sound production, food processing, and swallowing.

The presence of bones within our soft tissues provides passive support to our long limbs and reduces the amount of muscle effort spent to hold us up—without the bones' support, there would need to be a huge amount of squeezing! However, biology always requires a cost-benefit compromise, and a significant cost of bone is reduced movement potential. Our limbs do not have the movement variability of an elephant's trunk, and bone shape, size, and alignment define and limit the directions in which movement takes place. But our leg muscles—and those of the elephant—are grateful for the extra internal support provided by the bones.

Each species has its own signature locomotor strategy and, even as children, we can mimic the full body expressions of many animals. We can differentiate the slink of a cat, the lumber of a bear, and the side-to-side amble of a crocodile. Without even thinking about it, we can morph our bodies to imitate each species—the tiptoe of a cat, the plantigrade bear, and the turned-out limbs of the crocodile with its cross-patterned walk. In each case, our movement imitation carries through our whole body as it adapts to the movement style.

Although each of us can demonstrate an inner appreciation of the body's interconnectedness without even thinking about it, textbook analysis is usually restricted to single joints and their movements.

One of the problems for texts has been to find a starting point. How does one begin to investigate the complexity of the body in movement—do we begin by looking at the skeleton and then the soft tissue? Or is it the soft tissue that drives the skeleton? Or are both the skeletal and muscular systems controlled by the all-powerful nervous system? Giving precedence—consciously or unconsciously—to isolated systems is fundamentally flawed and limits our perception and understanding. Our starting point should be the entire animal in the context of its environment.

Natural history museums are wonderful places to expand the intellectual limits imposed by our traditional education. Through their cleverly juxtaposed displays of the skeletal remains of various species we get a glimpse of the bound relationship between a species and its movement. Each species can be viewed in the context of its family group and evolutionary heritage, as well as the ecology in which it thrived.

> *There are some four million different kinds of animals and plants in the world. Four million different solutions to the problems of staying alive.*
> —**David Attenborough,** *Life on Earth*

Although we might think of an ecosystem in terms of its geographical position on the globe, ecosystems are also affected by altitude. Altitude and latitude can determine which species of tree can flourish. In the tree canopy, if fruit and nuts appear at the ends of taller branches, it helps to be small and lightweight to reach them. While heavier species are limited to accessing lower, stronger branches and must compete for more ground-based food.

The human body evolved with the same constraints. Our evolutionary history of genetic tweaks from vertebrate to mammal, quadruped to biped, has been further polished by ecological pressures. Today, through time and accident, we have escaped most ecological pressures by manipulating our environment and taking control of food production. However, we have not escaped the genetic history of our overall physiology. Our anatomy has changed very little in the last 300,000 years, and even less in the last few centuries since industrialization.

We have a body plan that developed many millennia ago for hunting and gathering. However, this hunter-gatherer body now lives in a modern technological world where the closest thing to hunting is trying to find our mobile phone behind the sofa. Very few of us now move enough to avoid being classified as

"sedentary." The offset between the body we evolved and the ecology we live in is a recipe for developing so-called *mismatch disorders*— our modern diet and movement habits no longer meet the expectations of our evolved physiology.[1] The prevalence of the resulting health conditions has led to a blossoming interest in functional medicine.

A functional approach to medicine uses lifestyle adaptations to counter the effects of lack of exercise, unhealthy diets, and our unchallenging environments. Our bodies are adapted for variety, but we live in a world of bland movement. Our homes, workplaces, and shopping malls are not only sterile in terms of their cleanliness, they are also sterile movement environments—they do not challenge our movement by pushing us much beyond a short jog to avoid the rain between the car park and the front door.

Exercise is one branch of functional medicine, and *functional movement* has been a recent trend within the fitness industry. As mentioned in chapter 1, it can be considered a branch of functional medicine really only if we understand the *why* and the *how*. One step toward that is to appreciate where we came from and why we have the movement abilities we possess. Then, not only can we move and exercise in better ways, we can also see full body movement in the context of where it came from.

------

[1]Mismatch disorders are health issues that arise because we live modern lifestyles (mostly diet and movement deficiencies) with a body evolved to cope with fresh, local, seasonal foods that require hunting or gathering. For more information see Daniel Lieberman's *Story of the Human Body* (Penguin, 2013).

Functional Anatomy and Tensegrity

If you want to teach people a new way of thinking, don't bother trying to teach them. Instead, give them a tool, the use of which will lead to new ways of thinking.

—R. Buckminster Fuller, *On the Wisdom and the Purpose of Life*

Over the last 20 years, the concept of tensegrity has become popular in movement and manual therapies, and it is an essential element for the visual appreciation of the reality of our movement. I have taught a tensegrity-based model of anatomy (figure 2.2) around the world for 20 years and have encountered many misunderstandings of

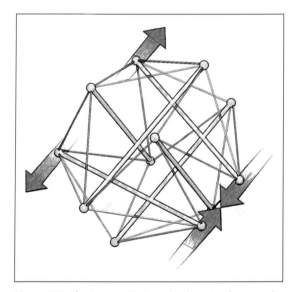

Figure 2.2. The tensegrity icosahedron is often used to show that the whole system reacts to any change in tension. This simplified presentation removes the variables of our anatomy with its joint alignments and restrictions alongside the multiple muscle and fascial fiber directions. (From Linus Johansson and Martin Lundgren, Movement Integration: The Systemic Approach to Human Movement *(Lotus, 2019)).*

anatomy because students are not made aware of the false assumptions within the standard anatomical model.

As already discussed, anatomical position has given us a limited image of the ways in which we move. When combined with traditional, simplified biomechanics, the reductionist teaching of the anatomical model has had a pervasive influence on our perception of human movement. Opening up to the reality of the body as a connected, interrelated, and interdependent entity can challenge some of the basics we thought we knew about the body, but the reality of interconnectedness would not have been a surprise if we started our study from observation of reality.

In contrast to the limitations of anatomical position, Gary Gray's "truth of movement" starting point is the observation of what is happening as someone makes a movement. I like this approach as it is based on *no expectations*—no rules, no theories, no instructions, no dogmas are applied. Just pure, unbiased observation.[2]

The job of a scientist is to listen carefully to nature, not to tell nature how to behave.

—Richard P. Feynman, *Classic Feynman: All the Adventures of a Curious Character*

Unbiased observation does not mean uninformed—this is not an excuse to throw away every anatomy book or, heaven forbid, to stop reading this text. Unbiased observation,

_____

[2]Although, as my colleague Owen Lewis would ask— even though we strive for unbiased observation, can we ever really achieve it?

for me, entails first identifying the movement strategy being used and then interpreting it from my understanding of real-life anatomy, and the starting position for that interpretation should be the acceptance of the body's interrelationships.

"It's all connected" has been a consistent message in movement and manual therapy training for many years, but we have had neither the clarity nor adequate vocabulary to describe and therefore understand what we see.[3] Our language skills for anatomy and the anatomy of movement have generally been those of separation, derived from the assumptions of the anatomical model. The "truth of movement" within a tensegrity structure is that when one part moves, the whole system responds and reacts. Now, we need to map out how and why it reacts in the way it does.

Too often, when learning a tensegrity approach to anatomy, one hears the idea that one change of tension could go *anywhere* through the body. While there are certain ways in which that may be true, it does little to empower us toward an understanding of how the body really responds during movement. In fact, to say the *whole* body responds and it *could go anywhere* is even less empowering for us than the original narrow anatomical model.

There is a middle path between these two extremes of the controlled, isolated traditional anatomy and the loose approach of tensegrity. Both extremes have useful elements of truth within them—there are measurable and dissectible units within the body, and they react in the context of the whole. We will benefit from understanding the details of anatomy *and* the wider contextual view of tensegrity.

---

[3]Until now!

The Predictability of Movement

Getting a few principles in place will help build a bigger picture from the jigsaw pieces of anatomy and tensegrity as we progress through the text. We will continually zoom out and in to see the big picture and its detail. But first let's start with an example of what I mean.

Stand up in a comfortable neutral position with your right hand lifted in front of you and keep looking at your right hand as you take it around to the right (figure 2.3). Go as far as you can and pause at the end of your range of movement.

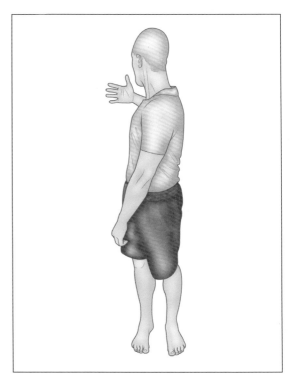

Figure 2.3. Turning to the right as your eyes and head follow the path of your right hand causes a repeatable predictable response through the body.

Take note of two things: (1) where your hand is pointing and (2) the changes in your feet. Can you feel that your left foot has pronated from where it started while the right foot has supinated?

Well, they *should* have.[4] If you turned as far as you can comfortably turn to your right, there is a reasonably predictable reaction through your whole body, a reaction that is determined by your anatomy. The reaction should have created not only pronation and supination at your feet but also a medial rotation of your right hip, a lateral rotation at your left hip, and an extension and rotation to the right of your spine. This is not the full list of predictable reactions to this movement, but they will suffice for now as we have much to learn before we can put the whole thing in context.[5]

There are two things we can do with the information from the exercise above—analyze why the predicted reactions happened or analyze why they did not. The rest of the book will reveal many of the reasons why our system responds the way it does, and—as therapists—it is also interesting and informative to understand some of the reasons why it might not.

Most therapies aim to identify and deal with areas that seem inconsistent with an expected or "normal" reaction during movement. Orthopedic assessments have given physical therapy wonderful tools to isolate areas of interest. Using specific and precise tests, dysfunctional joints and tissues can be diagnosed and the correct intervention applied. However, these anatomical-position-based tools go only a certain way toward dealing with the whole body and the way in which the client manages movement passing through their system.

As we saw in the exercise above and in figure 2.3, our whole body responds to the reach of one hand—therefore, we need an understanding of why that happens and what *should* happen during that movement (and to be able to predict what should happen during any movement). Therapists want to assist their clients and students toward a better relationship with their body by working toward comfortable, easy, appropriate, and full-body responses to movement. We are helping them toward some form of *integration* with their body.

What Is Integration?

Integration is a basic law of life; when we resist it, disintegration is the natural result, both inside and outside of us. Thus, we come to the concept of harmony through integration.
—**Norman Cousins**

Once, when I was assisting a structural integration class, a student asked, "What is meant by *integration*?" The lead teacher didn't provide a satisfactory answer, but instead was full of equivocations and obfuscations—mostly because *integration* in terms of anatomy and movement is difficult to define. I have struggled with that question ever since and the best that I can offer is:

---

[4] The reality is there are no hard **shoulds**, but there are strong expectations of what a "normal" reaction is.
[5] If you experience any confusion with the bone and joint descriptors do not panic—they will be explored and explained in chapter 8.

Integration is the whole body appropriately responding to any movement unless inhibited from doing so.

There are a couple of weasel words in there—how much or little response is "appropriate"? And what would "inhibit" the movement?

This book lays out the common, and therefore "appropriate," reactions to a range of movements. Seeing, understanding, and describing those reactions is a precious skill and is the main focus of this text. Like any skill, it is one that needs practice, and the learning process is helped by the predictability of our movement responses. Unlike the random tensegrity icosahedron, our anatomy—with its lumps and bumps, grooves, alignments, and even misalignments— still manages to provide some degree of predictability of movement reactions.

Hopefully you felt some of that predictability in the exercise above—you turned to the right and your left foot pronated while the right foot supinated. However, your reaction to the simple arm movement might have fallen into the "nonstandard" category.

Why do you think that might be?[6]

There are a few obvious options:

> **Environment:** Shoes, clothes, chairs, and workstation can all inhibit movement.
> **Injury history:** Current aches and pains and the protective responses learned from previous injuries can all affect your body's motor control response to help avoid

---

[6] I can't tell from here …

further aggravation. This type of response can last far beyond any actual need for protection as the body trains itself to avoid pain.
Beliefs: Unlike the unconscious reactions above, sometimes we consciously avoid certain movements, or we are taught "correct ways" to move. We should investigate where our (and our clients') movement beliefs come from.

Of course, there could be other options, and each reader, each client, or student might present new and novel reasons why their system doesn't respond in quite the way we might expect.

Identifying a client's movement strategy is a vital part of an assessment and treatment plan. This book will give you the language and therefore the visual skills to identify what is happening—or not—during a movement. Without that clarity, any plan will be handicapped, limited in its potential for success. The exercises and vocabulary in this text are designed to let you see anatomical relationships and their responses during movement and give you a strong guide toward successful treatments.

Movement Hierarchy and Kinetic Chains

Trust only movement. Life happens at the level of events, not of words. Trust movement.

—Alfred Adler

Human movement could be discussed from a variety of angles, each focusing on a different tissue or level of organization. The conscious and unconscious nervous system has significant influence on our movement abilities and restrictions. The nervous system can also direct muscle activity, tuning muscle tone, or adjusting their force output, and would be a suitable topic for many tomes. Our focus here will remain with the skeletal and soft tissue systems, and although we will pay particular attention to the soft tissue, it is the skeletal alignments that really create the predictability of our movement.

Knowing each bone's shape and size and its alignment with its neighbors provides us with a tool to understand how movement passes through the body. It was the skeletal arrangement around your ankle, between the malleoli and the talus, that caused your feet to pronate and supinate as you turned in the exercise above. That arrangement is almost universal from one human to the next because we all share the same vertebrate, mammalian, and primate lineage.

The skeleton is not the primary controller of movement—an argument could be made that the nervous system dictates what movements can or cannot be done—but the bones and their joints do form the outer boundaries of how far we can go in any given movement. For example, we might want to abduct the tibia to increase the valgus angle at the knee, but the ligaments around the knee joint would probably complain, because the arrangement of bones and ligaments at the knee is perfect for flexion and extension and limited in other directions.

A key to understanding functional anatomy will be the appreciation of the "movement grooves" and the "movement blocks" through the body's joints. Some joints, like the knee, will move easily in flexion and extension but resist rotation, while others—like the hip—might relish rotation but have limits in extension. Knowing each joint's movement tendencies improves our ability to track how movement passes through the body from one area to the next and gives us the power to predict the reaction in tissues far from the initial movement.

You experienced that power in the exercise above—you turned to the right and your right foot supinated and your left foot pronated. The predictability of the reaction in the feet is because our joints are not icosahedrons with potential to move in almost any direction—each joint has its particular ranges and limitations. Knowing the body part that is moving and the direction in which it moves is enough to know, more or less, what should happen in the rest of the body.

We have common, almost universal, full-body movement patterns. Although individuals vary in how they might walk, run, or throw, the basic strategy for each movement will be similar. Almost everyone will walk and run with a contralateral pattern, almost everyone will extend their spine to throw something. Each movement creates a predictable response in the soft tissues as the movement is channeled, or directed, through the body in ways that are determined by the movement grooves and blocks of the joints.

Everyday and sporting movement patterns reveal how full-body movement relates to the organization of our body and its anatomy. We will see the collaborative fiber directions from one muscle to the next, some of which might form myofascial continuities and many that don't. What is important is not tissue continuity but continuity of movement control through the body's sequenced chain of reaction.

It is not magic and there is no mystery. It is my intention to demystify the rather vague notion that "it's all connected" so we can grasp the basics of the interrelationship between movement direction, joint alignments, and soft tissues. We will then put in place the final piece of the puzzle by being clear with how to describe movement and tissue reactions.

Going Back to Go Forward

You cannot connect the dots looking forward; you can only connect them looking backwards.

— **Steve Jobs, "Connect the Dots" speech**

Understanding—really understanding—any subject begins with a firm grasp of the basics. There is always the temptation to jump ahead and try to delve into the complexities, because that makes us feel good about ourselves (if we can understand them, that is). However, we can soon get in over our heads. The learning process is easier, quicker, and more rewarding if a solid foundation is in place from the start. One of our main sources for understanding human movement is evolutionary anatomy.

Much insight into our overall body plan can be gained from evolutionary and comparative anatomy. These disciplines give context to the timing of evolutionary changes and help build a picture of what climate, migratory, and tool-use patterns existed before and after anatomical adaptations occurred. We can therefore start our learning process by first

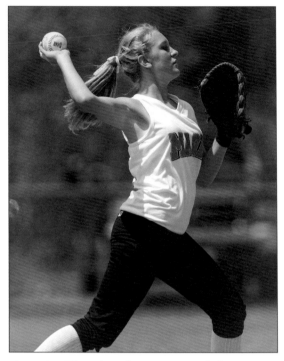

Figure 2.4. There have been many evolutionary changes to the human shoulder complex through time, but one of the most significant benefits for throwing was the development of lumbar extension.

taking a step backward, both figuratively into our past and literally by stepping back.

When we need more power, we often start by going backward. Think about how you throw and kick balls. Both movements start by going backward, and the more power you need, the further you tend to go back—but why do we do this? The answer lies in a relatively recent development in the physiology of our tissues.[7]

Look at the pitcher in figure 2.4. What is she throwing the ball with? We could break down the movement and analyze it in many

---

[7]In terms of evolution, two million years is quite recent.

ways, and I am sure we could use different vocabularies to do so. However, I hope that most of us could agree that she is using her whole body and not just the muscles around the right shoulder—an ability that is almost uniquely human, which, about two million years ago, was not present in our evolutionary lineage.

Homo erectus wandered onto the African landscape two million years ago and is generally regarded as the first of our ancestors to possess relatively modern human anatomy. One of the most significant features of *H. erectus* is its long waist; previous *Homo* species had very little space between the pelvis and rib cage. Even the very agile present-day apes have retained a relatively fixed relationship between the ribs and pelvis. We can see how the ape torso acts mostly as

one unit when we observe its gait because it lacks lumbar extension, which, frankly, makes apes even worse salsa dancers than me.

Our salsa dancing prowess is all thanks to the first *H. erectus*. The evolution of a longer waist—with increased lumbar movement that allowed the pelvis to move relatively independently of the rib cage—created new movement potentials for our ancestors. Communication of force through the whole body from extension into flexion was enhanced by an "uncoupling" of the thorax and pelvis.

Whether you salsa dance or not, almost everyone has tried to keep a Hula-Hoop spinning around their waist. We keep our ribs quite stable as we frantically gyrate our pelvis in synchrony with the turn of the hoop. If we

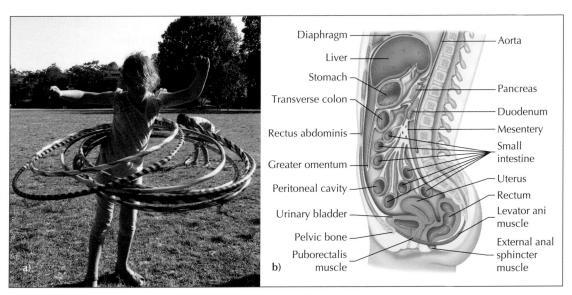

Figure 2.5. (a) Our mobile waist requires muscular control and myofascial support and has similarities with the muscular hydrostat arrangements of our tongue, elephant trunks, and octopus tentacles. (b) Three muscle layers with alternating fiber directions encompass a fluid-filled cavity encased between the respiratory and pelvic diaphragms. The abdominal muscles can therefore control both intra-abdominal pressure and direction of movement between the ribs and pelvis. (From Thomas Myers and James Earls, **Fascial Release for Structural Balance** *(Lotus, 2018)).*

consider the relationship between the ribs and pelvis as a joint, it has almost universal directionality, just like the muscular hydrostats we discussed above. Is it a coincidence that the fluid-filled abdomen is surrounded by three layers of muscle oriented in alternate directions, along with fascia and interstitial fluids, and encased between the respiratory and pelvic diaphragms (figure 2.5)?

Although the trend of the "abdominal core" is falling out of favor, it is still a useful concept to keep in mind. The problem with the "core" story that was so popular through the 1990s and into the early 2000s is that—like so many others—it was overhyped and overfocused on an isolated area. However, the general concept of stability and movement being adjusted by altering intra-abdominal pressure remains correct.

Rather than reducing down to the textbook stories about transversus abdominis and its connections, we should see the abdominal system in context of overall movement. We can then ask ourselves how does the abdominal area respond during movement? How does the whole body respond? What is the purpose of the abdominal area, and how does it react as movement passes between the pelvis and the rib cage?

We think of the lumbars as large, solid vertebrae with limited motion between the individual bones, but, cumulatively, between the sacrum and thoracic spine, we have a considerable range of movement. It was this increased movement between the ribs and pelvis that opened new and exciting movement possibilities for our *Homo erectus* ancestors. Greater spinal extension lets us stand straight and walk upright; allows us to throw, kick, and run with more power and efficiency; and

gives us the variability of movement that goes some way to making us human.

It is only anatomy books that consider the ranges of intervertebral motion to be important—our moving bodies are more interested in the "joint" between our pelvis and rib cage. We know that movement ability is produced by a collection of joints, and we should consider the whole body in the same way. The human body is a cooperative collective of joints that determine movement possibilities. Some joints are tightly bound and their movement groove is mostly predetermined, therefore their reactions are predictable. Other areas, such as the abdomen, have more variability. The one thing all joints have in common is that their movement potentials are created and controlled by myofascial patterning.

Myofascial Patterning

To understand is to perceive patterns. To make intelligible is to reveal the basic pattern.
—Isaiah Berlin, *The Proper Study of Mankind: An Anthology of Essays*

We will return to this subject in more detail later in the text, but for now it is useful to point out the correlation between joints and the soft tissues that cross them. Our muscle fibers can be arranged in a variety of patterns, such as the triangular arrangement around the hip or the more linear pattern either side of the elbow (figure 2.6). The reason for this becomes clear when you look at the moving body—each joint type has an associated soft tissue arrangement that makes sense when global movements are put in context.

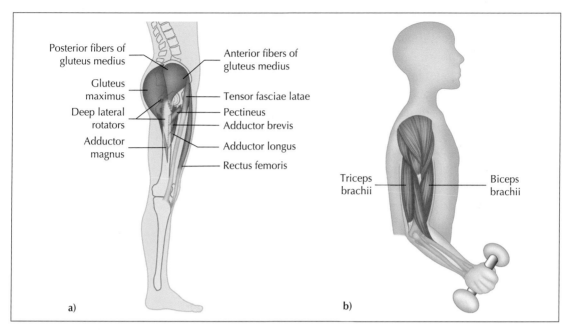

Figure 2.6. (a) Ball-and-socket joints, such as the hip and glenohumeral joints, require triangular muscle arrangements. (b) Having a wide range of muscle fiber directions would be redundant on a hinge-like joint such as the elbow.

Return your attention to the pelvic–rib-cage joint, which is spanned by an omnidirectional array of muscles. The rectus abdominis and erector spinae control flexion/extension, while the obliques and quadratus lumborum take care of rotation and side flexion. Each muscle can contribute to other actions, but the general pattern is easy to appreciate—the wide range of joint ability must be covered by an equally wide range of muscle fiber direction.

The same is true of ball-and-socket joints—their wide range of motion requires a complete array of soft tissues. For example, the body's two main ball-and-socket joints are surrounded by triangular arrangements of muscle, something that is redundant for hinge-like joints such as the elbow (figure 2.6).

Possibly the most important aspect to remember from this section and a key to appreciating the anatomy of movement is the correlation between joint type and soft tissue arrangement. Any motion that is available at a joint has to be controlled by the soft tissue, and the wider the range of motion, the wider the angle of muscle fiber will be required.

Read that paragraph again. It is really important.

Levers and Leverage

Men are moved by two levers only—interest and fear.

—Napoleon Bonaparte,
In His Own Words

You may have noticed that I have referred to "hinge-like" joints above. I make that adjustment from "hinge" to "hinge-like" in response to the current trend of challenging the language of anatomy. Analyzing the meaning, intention, and implications of words is extremely important and a very useful exercise—language, by its nature, provokes images of what things look like. Our joints do not resemble mechanical hinges except in their preferred direction of movement.

Our "hinge" joints do have some degree of motion, or "joint play," in directions beyond simple flexion/extension—perhaps you have experienced some doors like that? Our goal here is to create a global view and understanding of movement that allows us to see and assess individuals in movement. Within that we have to recognize that language is here as a tool toward that learning—sometimes we will benefit from pedantry and sometimes sticking to absolutes will get in the way.

One of the reasons for moving away from using the term "hinge joint" is because, unlike a mechanical hinge, there is no single fixed point around which movement occurs. A wider implication is that there can therefore be no *levers*. Levers are a common tool used by biomechanists in their analyses of movement, especially for measuring force and power output—however, this concept and use of language is objected to by many in the tensegrity field. You will be glad to know that we do not have to revisit our physics skills, but we should dig a little deeper to understand the difference between *levers* (rigid members rotating around a fixed point) and *leverage* (how limb length, for example, can influence force production).

The joint movements that we call flexion and extension generally give us the largest ranges

of motion—think of your elbows, knees, and spines. Each of those joints provides a lot of relatively free movement. While no joint acts as a pure lever, both the length of the bones and the length of our body contribute toward leverage, which can provide more force for individual movements. Importantly, it is not any single joint that provides the leverage, rather the accumulated range through a number of joints.

Before two million years ago, our ancestors had longer upper limbs and shorter lower limbs as a hangover from an earlier tree-dwelling species. Moving around and in between trees did not require an upright stance, and the ability to balance was probably enhanced by having short, flexed lower limbs (figure 2.7).

As we spent more time on the ground and harvested the benefits of an upright stance, there was greater impetus toward improved movement efficiency and getting our head above our straighter lower limbs. Increasing the range of motion through our lumbar spine came with other secondary benefits, because we could now extend through our entire body and increase our overall range of movement. Not only could we get our head almost directly above our feet, but the body's increased range of movement helped lengthen our stride (figure 2.8), our overhead reach, and our backward reach for those throws we looked at earlier (see figure 2.4).

Orthopedic-based anatomy has drawn our attention to the importance of *range of motion* for each joint and within each range. While it is extremely useful to assess and monitor individual joint range, it is also informative to consider the body's overall *range of movement*.

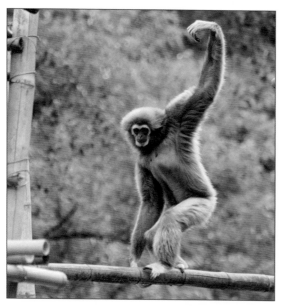

Figure 2.7. Although apes can walk upright, they do so with flexed hips and knees—but that is not because they cannot extend those joints. Apes have to keep their lower limbs flexed to help bring their torso over their feet because they cannot extend their spines enough. The knee and hip flexion is a compensation for lack of spinal extension.

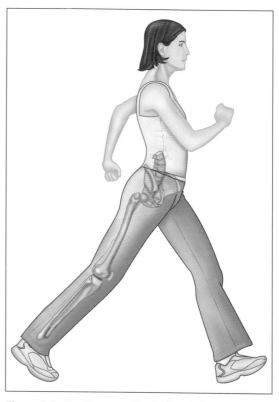

Figure 2.8. Our increased spinal mobility allows for longer strides (though that stride length is also made up of a series of joint extensions and quite a lot of rotation).

Our stride length and the cocking phase for a throw are particular examples of how our overall body plan has allowed for increased distance between supporting and working limbs. In gait, the supporting back leg helps propel the working leg forward, and in throwing, the anchored front and back feet provide a solid platform for the throwing arm. The distance between these points helps recruit more soft tissue into the movement by creating a continuity of strain through much of the body.

Causing the tissues to strain provides a number of benefits for force production and movement efficiency, which we will explore in chapter 3. For now, we simply need to see how

movement travels through the whole body. The communication of force, particularly seen in the throwing action, is made possible only by our mobile waist. The extension and rotation—made possible by the lumbar joints and controlled by the abdominals and intra-abdominal pressure—allow us to take advantage of greater leverage through our whole body.

"There is no such thing as a lever in the body" is a common refrain in tensegrity forums. They are correct—no joint has a precise, hinge-like, single axis action—but every joint has some movement in other planes because a joint's point of rotation might change as the bones move; and muscles do not work in the simplified and outdated idea of agonist-antagonist pairings. We can still apply the principles of *leverage*, however, to appreciate the effects of bone length and limb ratios on overall ranges of movement.

The evolutionary change toward longer lower limbs helped us lengthen our stride for walking and running, just as the gibbons increased their upper limb length to improve the efficiency of their brachiation (figure 2.9a). We then devised ways to compensate for our relatively shortened upper limbs—we invented "arm extending" devices (figure 2.9b and c), and, importantly, we increased the overall range of countermovement by developing the pelvic-rib-cage "joint" discussed above.

Tying It All Together

Compare the bodies of the pitcher and the gibbon in figures 2.4 and 2.9a, respectively. The gibbon's shoulder and body seem as if they are quite separate units—the trunk is swinging under the arms—whereas the pitcher is using her whole body to help her throw. There is a connection and interaction through the human system that appears to be missing in the gibbon. We might not be as fast or elegant as we clamber from branch to branch, but our ability to communicate force through our body enhances the adaptability of our movement—the human body is not as strong or as fast as the ape's—but we can swim, climb, jump, hop and skip, throw, and crawl.

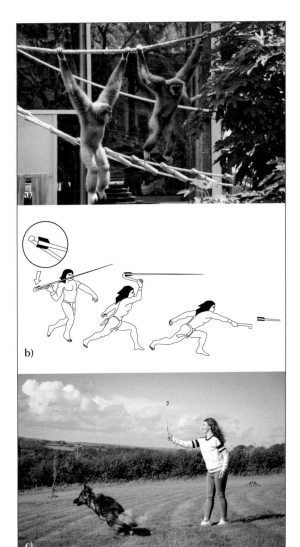

Figure 2.9. (a) Longer upper limbs help gibbons swing fast (note their flat backs!) and with more efficiency. (b) Humans have invented a variety of tools to compensate for our shorter arms and increase leverage for a throw. (c) You can still see a version of the atlatl (ancient Mexican throwing-stick) every day in your local park.

There is strong evidence that our modern shape (so-called "anatomically modern human") came about owing to the survival benefits of long-range walking, persistence hunting, and throwing. Each of these three movement patterns uses a different strategy or anatomical arrangement. The efficiency of long-range walking is as a result of a straight leg gait, while ultradistance running is best done with a flexed hip and knee, and throwing benefits from a full body extension. I think this variety of movement is a major key to our success as a species.

The long, narrow waist that helped us stand upright created new and exciting movement possibilities, especially the communication of force between the upper and lower body, by joining distant parts of the body. These connections and interactions occur at different angles and at different tissue levels and form useful avenues for control of movement and the production of extra force by using our whole body to enhance our mechanical advantage through leverage.

We have come to think of individual joints as levers, while a more useful concept is one of *leverage* through the whole body. Just as the dog walker is using the plastic ball-thrower, the pitcher is using her lower limb to help propel the ball forward. Seeing the body in this connected and interrelated way opens up new possibilities for defining the "actions" of individual muscles—is the rectus femoris a hip flexor and knee extensor, or is it a shoulder flexor? The pitcher's hip will extend during the preparatory cocking movement, putting energy into the tissue around the rectus femoris muscle that can then be used for the throwing action—making rectus femoris a contributor to shoulder flexion. Should we define a muscle only by the joints it crosses or by the movements it influences? The answer should be both.

We need to know the joints a muscle crosses, but we also need to widen our vision to appreciate how the whole body interacts in real-life movement. The first is a relatively straightforward, boring, and unsatisfying exercise in rote memorization, and the second is an initially difficult and complex task that is ultimately rewarding because it allows us to build the complete picture of human movement.

Summary

We are the facilitators of our own creative evolution.

—**Bill Hicks**

This chapter has explored the larger concepts of evolutionary and functional anatomy to demonstrate the origins of the human skeleton. There is a two-way relationship between the shape of the skeleton and the arrangement of the soft tissues that support it. Each available joint motion must have muscle fiber available to create and control that motion. Fiber direction, or muscle orientation, therefore, coincides with movement direction at each joint.

There are certain areas that have wider ranges of motion. The ball-and-socket joints of the hip and shoulder are surrounded by complex, triangular arrangements of muscles, and our recently evolved mobile waist is supported by a series of layered tissues that act like the mobile hydrostatic mechanisms of elephant trunks and our own tongue.

Traditional anatomy considers the body one structure at a time, but our movement requires the immediate orchestration, coordination, and cooperation of the whole body. The vocabulary of tensegrity provides us with the necessary imagery to visualize the body as an interactive whole, while knowing anatomy provides us with the understanding of how movement can be predictable.

Knowing how most bodies *should* react, we can then use that knowledge to assess clients or students and apply appropriate interventions to help them move in a more integrated, comfortable, and efficient way.

Reflection Questions

1. How do you think the human body is well adapted to our current ecology, and which aspects of our anatomy or the environment are no longer matched?
2. What is your understanding of how tensegrity and the relative predictability of human movement interact?
3. What are the relationships between joint alignments and muscle fiber direction?
4. What is the difference between *levers* and *leverage*?
5. What is your definition of "integration"?

Notes and Recommended Reading

I find comparative anatomy develops a deeper appreciation of the "why": Why are we shaped like this? Why do we move like this? By comparing ourselves to other species, especially vertebrates, we open our vision to our place in the ecosystem and gain context for the abilities and limitations of our human anatomy. If you would like to take the study further, I recommend the popular science titles of Steven Vogel, Neil Shubin, and Daniel Lieberman as excellent starting points.

Anatomy, tensegrity, and biotensegrity: Quite a few works have been written about this new "biotensegrity" approach to anatomy, some of them better than others. As a young science it is developing rapidly and, at time of writing, suffers from the power struggles of a new science in the modern world of marketing and social media summaries. To gain a solid introduction I recommend the work of Stephen Levin (who first adapted the term), Graham Scarr, and Susan Lowell de Solórzano.

Coyne, J. A. *Why Evolution Is True*. Penguin Books, 2014.

Lieberman, D. *The Story of the Human Body*. Vintage Books, 2014.

Roberts, A. M. *The Incredible Unlikeliness of Being: Evolution and the Making of Us*. Heron Books, 2015.

Scarr, G., and S. M. Levin. *Biotensegrity: The Structural Basis of Life*. Handspring, 2018.

Shubin, N. *Some Assembly Required*. Oneworld, 2021.

———. *Your Inner Fish*. Vintage Books, 2014.

Solórzano, S. L. de. *Everything Moves*. Handspring, 2020.

3

Fascia—the Body's Problem Solver

Introduction

Life is a continuous exercise in creative problem solving.
—**Michael J. Gelb, *Brain Power: Improve Your Mind as You Age***

It is important to keep in mind that words are a dissection of reality.

As we have seen, traditional anatomy teaching gives the impression that we can understand the whole by understanding the parts and then using those parts to build the body back up. That cannot be done.

To understand the language of anatomy we must start from the whole body and put that gestalt into the context of movement. The complete, integrated body is the reality, and all the descriptors we use only provide inadequate allusions to its complexity. Any division of the moving body into systems serves us by providing some descriptive power over a few important dynamics. However, the myofascial, or any other, system does not exist independently and cannot be isolated—it is a constructed convenience that facilitates discussion.

Humans have numerous movement strategies to gain more speed and more force, one of which is to start a movement by going in the opposite direction. We saw this with the action of throwing in chapter 2—we use extension to gain more force through the flexion phase. Some of that increased force is due to the improved leverage, and some is because the countermovement pretensions the fascial tissues. These connective tissues have many properties that improve movement efficiency, especially when they are pretensioned.[1] This chapter provides a working introduction to these mechanisms and gives some suggested reading for further exploration.

---

[1] Fascia is one of many *connective tissues*. As I won't be discussing the other connective tissues (such as blood and epithelium), and as fascia is the connecting tissue through the body, I will use the two terms "fascia" and "connective tissue" synonymously.

The Problems—Like Finding a Title to a Section

There is no such thing as a problem without a gift for you in its hands.
—**Richard Bach, *Illusions***

We have already seen that biology always requires a cost-benefit compromise. Muscle fibers help us move, but they come with quite a few limitations. Muscle fibers provide movement control through their contractions (eccentric, concentric, and isometric) but they require a plentiful energy source consisting of sugars and proteins. Muscle fibers are also delicate and break easily under strain, strain that is often predictable but will sometimes come from a variety of angles. Not only are the muscle fibers delicate, but when they tension they operate best within only a small range of length and speed—they rapidly weaken when the fibers are too short, too long, or have to contract too quickly. Furthermore, our hunter-gatherer body would be too heavy and too calorie-consuming to survive if the only soft tissues were muscle fibers. Thankfully, the many forms of fascial tissue go some way to compensating for these potential weaknesses.

An array of fascial tissues that encapsulates the muscle fibers ameliorates each of the above issues (figure 3.1). Fascia not only provides a lightweight but strong scaffolding for force transfer to and from muscle fibers, it also helps improve muscle efficiency and balances out the potential weaknesses in muscle performance when the tissues change length or work at high speeds.

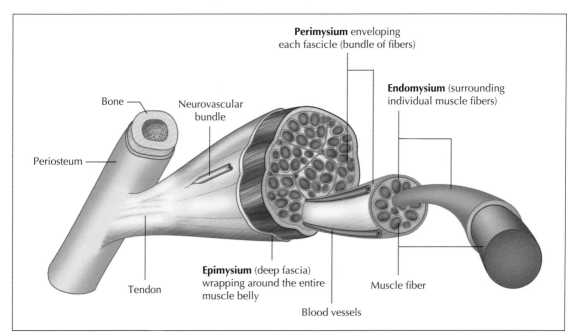

Figure 3.1. Collagen-rich fascial tissue envelops individual muscle fibers and bundles of them. Seen here as the endomysium, perimysium, and epimysium, these fascial "bags" provide scaffolding for muscle cells and many mechanical advantages. The combination of muscle and fascia—known as myofascia—*therefore provides support, assists force transfer, and enhances performance.*

We will focus mainly on the logic behind the hierarchical and complementary arrangement of tissue types. Details on the makeup and percentages of the various fascial strands are easy to find, and I have suggested further reading resources at the end of this chapter. Understanding the mechanisms used during our movement is more important for us at the moment.

Efficiency and Countermovement

It's not the most powerful animal that survives. It's the most efficient.
—**Georges St-Pierre, FaceBook, May 25, 2011**

Many studies have shown how fascial tissue can act as a spring to help reduce the metabolic costs of movement—a useful benefit for survival in our evolutionary past. Fewer calories are used if muscle fibers remain close to isometrically contracted while the body uses gravity, momentum, and ground reaction forces to lengthen the elastic fascial tissues. Collagen fibers within the myofascia can then recycle much of the energy used to stretch them, just like an elastic band will recoil with energy after being drawn into a stretch.

To appreciate how active countermovement works, it helps to see the difference between actively and passively strained tissue (figure 3.2a) and what is meant by "stretch." In most cases, we use "stretch" when we should use the term "strain." In common usage, "stretch" is loosely and poorly defined, and there is much debate as to what it actually means and what is actually happening when we *stretch* tissue.

Officially, the *stretch* of the collagen fiber is known as *strain*, which is the measurement of how much the tissue has deformed. Although commonly seen as a change in length, strain can refer to a change in any dimension—something that is important to keep in mind, as we see only two dimensions on the printed page. When a muscle is eccentrically contracting, it increases not only in length but can also increase in width and in depth. We frequently measure myofascial strain as a change in length, but compare the images in figure 3.2a—a passive stretch of the tissue simply lengthens it— an eccentric, active loading of myofascial tissue causes the tissue to expand in every direction, a feature of some biological tissues known as *auxeticity*.[2]

The auxetic nature of myofascia helps disperse eccentric loading forces in every direction rather than focusing them between the polar ends of a muscle. Myofascia wraps around individual muscle fibers, bundles of fibers, and the whole muscle, effectively intertwining it and making it part of its structure. Because of this, its three-dimensional structure can be strained in every direction, more like a balloon than an elastic band (figure 3.2b). This means that fascial containment of fiber bundles improves muscle force output, as the containment creates a stiffened environment that transfers muscle force more effectively and efficiently.

---

[2] Changes in tissue dimension under strain are measured according to a simple formula known as Poisson's ratio. If you would like to understand more about auxeticity and tissue expansion, I recommend a simple internet search.

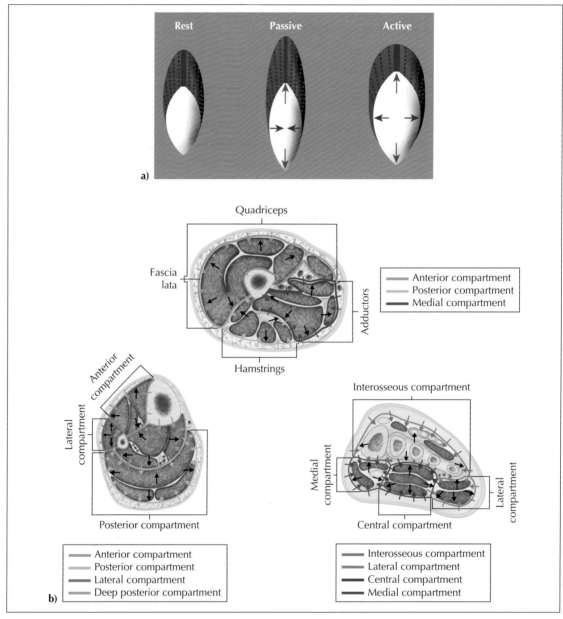

Figure 3.2. (a) A myofascial unit (i.e., a muscle fiber and its supporting fascia) is lengthened during a passive stretch, but the unit acts differently when it is actively lengthening. As the muscle fibers contract eccentrically to decelerate movement, the overall volume of the muscle increases and the myofascial unit expands in each dimension. (b) Myofascial expansion and auxeticity during eccentric work accounts for the body's propensity for muscle compartments. The body uses a reciprocal arrangement between tensioning compartments (through movement and muscle attachments to the sheaths) to compress the muscles and uses the expansion of the contained muscles to tension the compartment sheaths. ((a) is based on T. J. Roberts and E. Azizi, "Flexible Mechanisms: The Diverse Roles of Biological Springs in Vertebrate Movement," Journal of Experimental Biology *214 (2011): 353–61).*

Our movement naturally exploits that fact by preparing for most actions by first going in the opposite direction. To continue with the example of throwing, it is the body's flexors that will be recruited to produce most of the force into the projectile as the arm goes back. A summary of those flexors would include rectus abdominis, rectus femoris, the psoas, and iliacus, along with the anterior adductors of the back leg and, of course, pectoralis major. Each of these muscles has to work to decelerate extension during the preparatory cocking, and this active eccentric muscle contraction creates lengthening and expansion of the fascial tissues.

It is commonly thought that muscle fibers decelerate countermovement by staying close to isometric, which keeps them within their optimum force-length ratio. This idea is a simplification of the force-length curve seen in many textbooks (figure 3.3a). A number of researchers have shown that muscle fibers adjust their length-tension ratio to work on the so-called "ascending limb" of the curve (figure 3.3b). Muscle sarcomeres change their length in response to the forces acting through them—the higher the force, the shorter they will become. The result is that when muscles have to work eccentrically, they are moving toward the peak of the force-length curve.

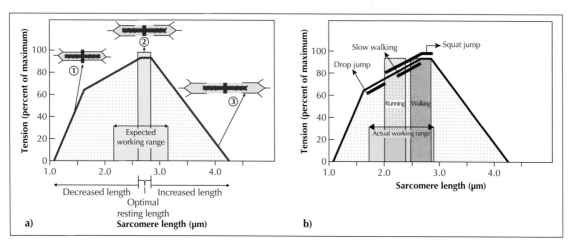

Figure 3.3. (a) Sliding filament theory and many measurements show that muscle fibers produce less force when they are too short (labeled "1") or too long (labeled "3"). When the fibers are too short, the actin and myosin filaments overlap and inhibit further contraction. When the fibers are too long, the actin and myosin filaments have less overlap and fail to fully engage for contraction. It is usually thought that muscles operate optimally across the peak of the force-length curve ("2"). (b) A proprioceptive feedback loop lets a muscle fiber calibrate its length to optimize its ability to control eccentric movement. When external forces are higher, such as during running, the sarcomere length is reduced to give more leeway for the fiber lengthening that occurs during the eccentric phases. By recalibrating itself, the muscle becomes more efficient and helps protect the tissues by reducing the possibility of going over the peak of the force-length curve and becoming too weak to control the eccentric movement. The operating range is now adjusted to fully focus along the ascending limb of the curve and does not cross over the peak of the curve. The readjustment allows the muscle fiber to lengthen without handicapping its ability to create force—it remains strong. (Based on M. Ishikawa, J. Pakaslahti, and P. V. Komi, "Medial Gastrocnemius Muscle Behavior during Human Running and Walking," **Gait and Posture** 25, no. 3 (2007): 380–84).

These findings show that the force-length curve is not fixed and that muscles use a feedback loop to reset their sarcomere length to optimize the system. That optimization allows muscles to become stronger as they lengthen during the eccentric phase of a movement and, despite lengthening, prevent the fiber length from going over the top of the force-length curve. If muscle fibers lengthen beyond the top of the curve, they rapidly weaken and are therefore less able to control the movement.

A fiber recalibrating its length to get stronger as it lengthens makes sense for tissue protection. Think of the difference between kicking a ball for a child to catch and propelling the same ball across a soccer pitch. When we need more force, we tend to go further toward the end of joint range—we get more leverage for the intended movement, but we also put ourselves in easily compromised positions (yet another example of cost/benefit). Thankfully, the body has more than one defense mechanism—as the tissues strain, lengthen, and expand they also become stiffer.

Tissue Stiffness and Stress

Stress should be a powerful driving force, not an obstacle.
—**Bill Phillips,** *Body for Life: 12 Weeks to Mental and Physical Strength*

As with stretch and strain, tissue stiffness and stress are also commonly confused dynamics, mostly because of the various other ways in which we use the two terms "stiffness" and "stress" in everyday language. Take a moment and follow the exercise in figure 3.4 to get the sense of what happens as you move your finger toward its end of range.

The finger gives little resistance during the early stages, but, as you will have found, we have to pull much harder as the tissues get longer and the joint moves toward its end of range. The tissue is therefore less stiff when it is short and becomes stiffer as it lengthens.

This is the simplest explanation I have found. There are many formulae and official definitions if you wish to delve further into tissue dynamics. There is also a fancy graph

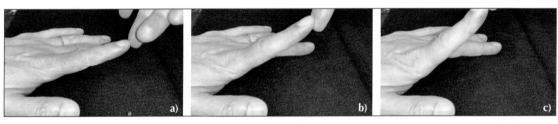

Figure 3.4. (a) Rest your nondominant hand on the table as shown, and use the other hand to pull the index finger upward a short distance. Before you feel any sense of a "stretch," release the index finger and let it fall. Note the sound it makes as it hits the surface. (b) Now repeat the same movement, but take the index finger back to where you feel a "stretch" and let go. Notice the sound it makes as it hits the surface. (c) This time bring your finger back to where it almost hurts, and then release and note the change in sound. Repeat the exercise, noting the resistance you feel from the index finger—the further into extension it moves, the more it resists.

below but, be warned, graphs can sometimes cause more confusion than clarity if you are not used to them. If the example in figure 3.4 makes sense and graphs make you nervous, just skip the section below (you won't miss that much—but you will miss out on why the sounds changed when you let go of your finger …).

Vocabulary Builder

Resistance to lengthening is referred to as *stiffness*.
Lengthening of the finger flexor tissue is referred to as *strain*.
The amount of force you had to apply to overcome the tissue's stiffness as the strain increased is known as *stress*.

To summarize—you applied more *stress* to overcome increased tissue *stiffness* as the tissue *strained*.

(The Part You Can Skip Over if Graphs Are a Mystery)

> *In my perception, the world wasn't a graph or formula or an equation. It was a story.*
> —**Cheryl Strayed**, *Wild: From Lost to Found in the Pacific Trail*

Ms. Strayed was partially correct: life is not a graph and it's best described in stories. But a good graph also tells a story when you know how to interpret it. You will see similar graphs in every biomechanics book, but they rarely tell the story to help you put it in context. So, sit back and let us begin …

In biomechanics, the force you applied to stretch your finger to pull it back is referred to as *stress*. By pulling your finger back you applied a stress to the flexor tissues, and the stress caused the soft tissues to change in length and breadth. The changes to the soft tissue can be measured and are referred to as *strain*.

The energy of the stress (the pull from one finger) causes the flexor soft tissues (on the finger being pulled) to strain, and as they strain those tissues also capture and store energy. You can feel and hear that energy by simply letting go at the end of each of the three "stretches"—the more strain on the tissues, the more energy is released when you let go (figure 3.5).

The stored energy is shown as shading on the graph and demonstrates to us two important dynamics (figure 3.5b). In the early part of the movement (shown as zone 1), the tissue lengthens along the horizontal axis (the *strain* measurement), but little energy is captured. More energy is captured in the second zone, where the tissue lengthens by an equivalent amount as in zone 1 (shown by the length along the horizontal axis) but we had to apply much more *stress* to achieve that length (shown by the height gain along the vertical axis).

We can put that into a three-dimensional image by thinking of the balloon again. As kids, most of us spent many hours blowing up balloons and letting them go. But our balloons never seemed to go as far or make as much noise as when an adult had blown them up. The stronger lungs of an adult can overcome more of the balloon's elastic resistance, strain it further, and thereby load more energy into it. That stored energy is then released and propels

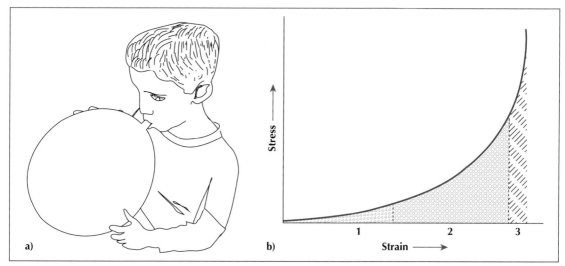

Figure 3.5. Transferring information from linear graphs to 3-D biological tissues can be difficult. As we saw in figure 3.2a, myofascial units expand in every dimension during eccentric contractions, kind of like a balloon (a). You felt how the flexor tissue increased its resistance as you lengthened it in the exercise in figure 3.4. Now we can put it all together in a graph (b). Natural materials have variable degrees of stiffness as they strain. In the early phase of lengthening (1), little stress is required and not much energy (shown as triangles) is loaded into the tissue during the strain. The situation, in terms of energy loading, is similar toward the end of lengthening (3), when the tissue becomes stiffer and therefore offers more protection to the joints. Here, more energy (stress) is required to lengthen (strain) the material and, because of the small degree of extra length (strain) gained, less energy is added for the return movement (hatched area). It is in the middle phase (2) where the most energy is loaded into the tissue for its return (shown in small circles).

Biological tissues alter in stiffness as they change size, in some ways like a balloon. Initially, putting air into the balloon is easy—it gives little resistance as it goes from floppy to a little taut (zone 1). Unlike biological tissues, the balloon's resistance to further inflation doesn't change much thereafter (zones 2 and 3), though we do feel as if we have to blow harder as the balloon reaches the limits of its capacity. Eventually, the balloon will burst, just as our tissues will tear if we overstrain them (beyond zone 3). Unlike the balloon, our tissues resist damage by increasing their stiffness as they lengthen.

the air outward—a kind of three-dimensional countermovement strategy.

Moving into the graph's second zone takes a little more input of stress (we go up the vertical axis much more) but it also captures more energy (the area with circles under the graph increases). That energy can then be recycled as elastic energy to assist with the return movement.

As we go further toward the third zone, we are getting toward the dangerous area of tissue failure and risk causing compromise to the joints. In this area we don't want to lengthen much more, we want to protect tissue integrity by making it more resistant to further strain.

(You can start reading here again if you wish—but you missed a bit about balloons!)

All change is not growth, as all
movement is not forward.

—**Ellen Glasgow**

Most everyday movements (typing, making a cup of tea, passing that cup across to your loved one …) generally require very little strain in the tissue. We normally work within the area of minimal resistance—it is rare that we stretch to turn on the kettle, or to reach the keys at the edge of the keyboard. Think about all the small movements you have made while reading this book so far—turning the page, maybe making some notes, or reaching for your cocktail. This inner movement range, represented by the first finger stretch in the exercise in figure 3.4 or zone 1 on the graph in figure 3.5b, is mostly controlled by short-range muscle actions. As we mentioned previously, muscle contractions are metabolically expensive (and require lots more graphs with even scarier chemistry!), but by staying in this short range, the muscles receive less resistance to their movement, making it easy and economical to perform repetitive everyday tasks.

Most sporting and exercise movements require high levels of force and, therefore, take us out of zone 1 and into the upper reaches of zone 2, where we capture more energy in the tissue by straining it further.[3] The easiest way to get that strain, load the energy, and then use it for the return movement is through countermovement. Going in the opposite direction first uses momentum to create tissue strain—think of the kicking or throwing examples mentioned earlier. We do not use a slow, controlled, mindful contraction of the "antagonist" muscles to load the pectoralis major for a throw, instead we almost whip our hand back. Or we swing our leg backward with some speed to prepare for a kick. While the concentric contraction of the antagonist muscles may be involved (e.g., to initiate a fast countermovement from a standing start), it is the momentum of the backswing that provides most of the stress required to strain the tissues enough to load the right amount of elastic energy.

But it is not all about elastic loading. Our inner proprioception guides us on how to adjust the necessary variables to create the right amount of power to achieve the desired outcome. Those variables include:

1. **Speed of the countermovement:** Experiment by throwing a scrunched-up piece of paper across the room, first with a fast and then with a slow countermovement. Faster countermovement creates more momentum and generally results in more force for the throw.
2. **The timing of the release:** Now try the same actions but pause at the end of the countermovement before throwing. The pause causes some loss of stored energy and increases *hysteresis*.[4]

---

[3] I should point out that the zones I have constructed are arbitrary and purely for illustrative purposes—this is not an official delineation. The reality of tissue stress and strain relationships and elastic loading is a three-dimensional continuum.

[4] Hysteresis is the fancy term for energy leakage from the system—not all of the energy used to load the elastic tissue is returned from it. Some energy is lost owing to friction and heat, or just disappears into the ether…

3. **The distance you move into the countermovement:** This is the obvious variable and is the one we learn through trial and error as children. If you want to throw or kick further, you make a longer countermovement. Going further back will:

   a. **Recruit more tissues:** Try throwing your piece of paper with just your arm instead of with your whole body, and observe the differences in force production.

   b. **Load more energy into the elastic tissue in preparation for the movement:** By going further into the stretch we move toward the end of zone 2 and possibly into zone 3. Creating more strain in the tissue captures more elastic energy—you might feel this as you lean back into the stretch.

   c. **Increase the leverage for the movement:** Again, think of the throwing action and how lumbar extension has allowed modern humans to use their whole body for more forceful movement.

Moving further into a countermovement—for most sporting-type actions—is a virtuous cycle. Longer countermovements achieve more leverage, recruit more tissues, and allow the capture of more energy. But there are dangers associated with the long lever positions created during high-force actions—we are more prone to breaking as they take us toward tissue limits. Thankfully, the myofascia is designed to increase its resistance to strain—it stiffens as it lengthens to help protect us as we move into challenging positions.

Eccentricity, Extensions, Elasticity, and Velocity

That so few now dare to be eccentric, marks the chief danger of the time.
—**John Stuart Mill, *On Liberty***

Once we have got into a lengthened position, the next step is to perform the action, and, usually, the further we have gone into the countermovement the more force we are planning to use. Now we have a new problem—muscle fibers are relatively weak when they contract concentrically at high speeds (figure 3.6).

Muscle fibers work differently at different speeds, depending on the direction of their contraction, and this is why biomechanists talk about force and velocity relationships. *Velocity* is speed of movement in a particular direction—in this case, concentric or eccentric. The physiology of muscle tissue means that muscles can produce more force as they *eccentrically* contract with more speed. But our intended action following the countermovement (to throw, kick, or jump) will require *concentric* contractions, and these produce less force when we contract quickly.

Thankfully, we do not have to rely solely on concentric muscle contraction for a forceful return movement. The countermovement has loaded plenty of elastic energy into the collagenous tissues and they can release that energy rapidly. As collagen tissues shorten the muscle fibers can also shorten, but at a lower velocity than the collagen fibers, which optimizes the combined force production.

But remember what we said about dissecting reality—we tend to think that the fascial tissues "compensate" for some of the limitations in muscle because we have been taught to think that we have *muscle* and we have *fascial tissue*, and the two are somehow separate. But they aren't. All vertebrates have an intricately blended series of cell and fiber types that cooperate to help us survive. The separate analysis of cell and fiber types helps us understand their roles, but we should always come back to the fact that we are complete, connected systems.

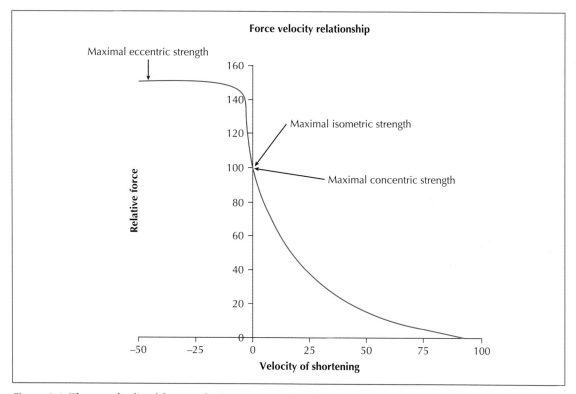

Figure 3.6. The standardized force-velocity curve can be a little confusing after looking at the stress-strain curve (figure 3.5b). The important difference is that the neutral muscle length is in the middle of the horizontal axis. Strangely, the muscle is getting longer as we move to the left (labeled "eccentric") and shorter as we move to the right (labeled "concentric"). Velocity is speed with a direction, and the directions in this case are eccentric and concentric—lengthening and shortening. Notice that the numbers either side of the "0" are the same. but negative going to the left, which is eccentric, and positive going to the right, which is concentric.[5] The important learning points from this graph are that concentric contractions get weaker with increased speed, while eccentric contractions get stronger as their speed increases.

---

[5] Yes, I would have put the labels the other way around as well, but, for some reason, this is the standard convention.

Long-Chain Movement and Long-Chain Tissues

Regard this body as a machine which, having been made by the hand of God, is incomparably better ordered than any machine that can be devised by man, and contains in itself movements more wonderful than those in any machine. … It is for all practical purposes impossible for a machine to have enough organs to make it act in all the contingencies of life in the way in which our reason makes us act.

—Rene Descartes,
Discourse on Method

Although often blamed for promoting the idea of the body as a machine, Descartes did say that the body is more complex and more wonderful than any man-made invention. A major issue for many people when they approach the study of biomechanics (a man-made invention) is its lack of "connection." Generally, biomechanics and anatomy excel at investigating the individual parts, but, as we have seen so far, most daily and sporting movements use a series of joints and tissues. We also move with tremendous variability, and it is this complexity that we seek to understand. Despite the mismatch between everyday movement and what is presented in anatomy books, many of us have tried to build the picture up from the anatomical bits to the complex whole that we see in front of us.

Historically, textbooks have provided us with only a limited picture, and this was frustrating. This lack of satisfaction was part of the reason for the success of Thomas Myers's "anatomy trains" concept when it was first published in 1997, and then in full book form by Elsevier in 1999. The "trains" drew the therapy world's attention to this new-fangled fascia thing and seemed to provide a more holistic, wider, full-body view of anatomy, spawning numerous programs of foam rolling, Pilates, and yoga-based exercise programs. Finally, it looked as though there was a new map that matched the full-body, long-chain, tensegrity experience that many practitioners had been experimenting with.

Myers, a student of Ida Rolf, developed the anatomy trains idea when asked to teach anatomy at the Rolf Institute and has since expanded the concept into his own approach to structural integration. I was a teacher of this approach until 2016, when I realized that even this apparently complex map is itself a simplification of normal movement, and learning the details of each "train" is a distraction from seeing the beauty within the continuous, interconnected complexity of our anatomy.

Myers's ideas, by his own admission, were not original. Various anatomists and practitioners had come up with other ways to map the body and its myofascial continuities, the most famous being Dutch anatomist and physiotherapist Andry Vleeming. Vleeming has spent decades developing and researching the level of connections between supposedly discrete tissues and the amount of force that can be transferred from one anatomical unit to another. There are numerous overlaps in the tracks put forward by Myers and Vleeming and others.

However, we must address the difference between tissue continuity and the ability to transfer force. For example, when we go into any long-chain back bend, we feel a stretch—the anterior tissues are strained by the position we are in. The reality of the body, as we discussed at the start of this chapter, is its continuity and integrity. Our starting position for analysis should be from human movement to anatomy. Long-chain extension through our body is a common position because of the many mechanical advantages it affords us. It does not matter if we can identify direct myofascial continuities or not—the reality of the body is that it is continuous, and it finds efficient strategies to control any movement pattern.

For example, if we look at the overall pattern of human gait there is a consistency in the use of extension from the big toe to the sternum, perhaps even through the spine to the head (see toe-off position in figure 3.7). In the toe-off position we can see the overall pattern of movement creates a consistent line of stretch through the body, as the trunk and pelvis progress over the top of the planted foot, so we have a continuity of force rather than fascial continuity. It is therefore of little surprise or, for our purposes, importance that during a comprehensive review study Doctor Jan Wilke stated that "no evidence exists for the superficial front line" (figure 3.7).[6]

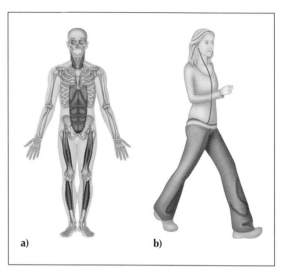

Figure 3.7. Various models of myofascial continuity have been put forward over the years. The best known is probably Myers's "anatomy trains," in which he proposes the "superficial front line" (a). Although no evidence exists for the superficial front line, we must accept that there is a corresponding overall extension pattern in much human movement (for example, in the toe-off position shown in b). The full-body extension pattern has to be controlled by tissues capable of managing the strains created and brings forth the question of whether we need myofascia to be continuous to manage force or simply capable of cooperating along the line of strain.

Linear myofascial continuity is not always involved with the production or control of movement. For example, when researching the connections between the biceps femoris and sacrotuberous ligament, Andry Vleeming found that the muscle transferred force to the ligament regardless of the amount of fascial connection (figure 3.8). Vleeming concluded that force could be transferred from the attachment site of the biceps femoris to the sacrotuberous ligament through "distortion of

———

[6] Jan Wilke, Frieder Krause, Lutz Vogt, and Winfried Banzer, "What Is Evidence-Based about Myofascial Chains: A Systematic Review," *Archives of Physical Medicine and Rehabilitation* 97, no. 3 (2016): 454–61.

the ischial tuberosity (bone elasticity)" rather than directly through the fascial tissues.[7]

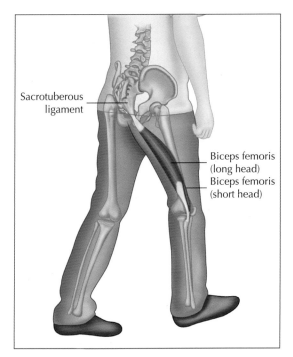

Sacrotuberous ligament

Biceps femoris (long head)
Biceps femoris (short head)

Figure 3.8. In 1993 Andry Vleeming and a small group of anatomists investigated the role played by the biceps femoris in movement and control of the sacroiliac joint. They found that all the subjects they dissected had continuity between the superficial fibers of both soft tissue elements, but 40% of them had no deeper connection and the ligament was "fully connected to the ischial tuberosity."[8] Despite this variation, force could be transferred from the biceps femoris to the sacrotuberous ligament in each condition.

[7] J. P. van Wingerden, A. Vleeming, C. J. Snijders, and R. Stoeckart, "A Functional-Anatomical Approach to the Spine-Pelvis Mechanism: Interaction between the Biceps Femoris Muscle and the Sacrotuberous Ligament," *European Spine Journal* 2, no. 3 (1993): 143.
[8] Ibid.

It appears that the influence of bone shape and joint alignment has been downgraded during the recent wave of interest in fascia. We must be mindful that each factor—tissue type, tissue properties, tissue architecture, and connectivity—plays a role in movement. We should highlight the problem with emphasizing anatomy over movement— too much time is wasted learning possible continuities instead of appreciating the "truth of movement."

Individual Variation

> *Always remember that you are absolutely unique. Just like everyone else.*
>
> —attributed to **Margaret Mead**

The variability of connection between the biceps femoris and the sacrotuberous ligament highlighted by Van Wingerden and Vleeming is a warning against basing any therapy on textbook anatomy. Anatomical variation is reported consistently in other papers which then serves as a reminder that there are no absolutes in anatomy—it is impossible to extend any finding to the whole population.

Remember to keep individual variations in mind as we progress through the exercises. We can expect certain reactions to happen because of the general human body plan, but we cannot hold everyone to that expectation. Although that might seem like a contradiction, it keeps us humble and alert as we try to unravel the mysteries that our clients sometimes present with. Through understanding the expected reactions to movement, we can begin to recognize the unexpected, because it is the unexpected reactions that draw our attention and potentially reveal clues from which we can begin to weave together the client's unique story.

The client is the expert on their own body. They might not know this yet, but their body holds many answers—our expertise lies only in trying to reveal what those answers might be. Our role is to guide them through a maze, encouraging them as they venture into unknown realms, and reassuring them that all is not lost if they come to an apparent dead end. Therapists and teachers can act like adventure guides, bringing each client along paths that may be unfamiliar to them both—but which are probably similar to ones the therapist has walked along before.

Learning to be a guide can also be daunting, because the reality of movement that we must face is its complexity. But we can learn to manage some of it through clarity of language and understanding. Just as any good explorer benefits from a grounding in geography, an appreciation of weather patterns, and an ability to work a compass, a seasoned guide to the body should be able to traverse any path with confidence. That is our goal here. We do not need to know every path nor every detail of each client's body and its abilities, nor could we as we don't have access to every scan and X-ray, let alone to every physical and emotional action and reaction they have experienced. Sufficiently prepared with a systematic vocabulary and a grounding in the principles, however, we can set off with confidence to safely explore and expand our clients' horizons—and our own.

Putting It Together—What Does It All Mean?

A Global Stretch-Shortening Cycle

1. Countermovement strategies are always used for any movement that requires extra force beyond the normal muscle contraction range (zone 1 in figure 3.5b).

2. Increasing the leverage for movement can increase the force, but that also increases the number of tissues and joints involved and moves them toward their end of range.

3. The soft tissues protect themselves by getting stiffer as they lengthen (zone 2 in figure 3.5b), and the muscles get stronger as they work eccentrically to control the cocking phase (going to the left of the graph in figure 3.6).

4. Especially during repeated actions, the muscle sarcomeres can adjust their length to optimize force control as they lengthen, preventing them from going too far over the top of the force-length curve (figure 3.3b).

5. Eccentric muscle force and stiffening of the tissues decelerate the cocking phase as the collagenous tissues strain (in all dimensions!) and capture elastic energy (the shading under the graph in figure 3.5b).

6. Captured elastic energy can then be released and used for the concentric movement (when the ball is finally kicked or thrown), and the rapid shortening of the strained fascial tissues compensates for the muscle tissues' loss of force during their rapid concentric contraction (going to the right of the graph in figure 3.6).

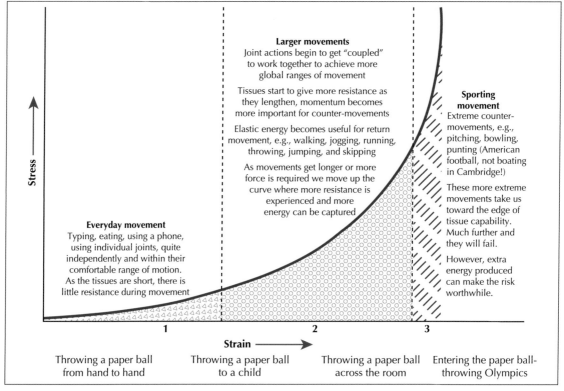

Figure 3.9. *The sliding scale of strain—the lengthening along the bottom of the graph—can be seen in the continuum from our small everyday movements through to the extreme forces needed for sport. The more force we need for a movement, the further we strain fascial tissues for all of the advantages they will offer us. Please keep in mind that the zones are only figurative and do not actually exist, they are a convenience to assist our understanding.*

The amalgamation of these dynamics is sometimes referred to as the "stretch-shortening cycle." The stretch produced by the countermovement helps increase force during the shortening phase (figure 3.9). Although most research and commentary on the stretch-shortening cycle focuses on sporting actions, countermovement and the benefits gained from it will occur any time we move into the (imaginary) zone 2 range of movement.

Using the Idea of Zones to Help See Tissue Contribution in Long-Chain Movement

Soft tissues are more efficient when their length and their velocity match the demands of the task. We cannot produce the force needed to win the paper-throwing Olympics without going toward end of range, and going to end of range would be unnecessary, and quite inappropriate, for throwing anything to a child.

When we come to analyze long-chain movements, all the soft tissue areas along the line of strain should match in their level of contribution—we do not want isolated areas being forced toward the outer extremes of zone 3 because other areas are still in zone 1, especially for strong and repeated sporting actions.

Unless, of course, there is a particular biomechanical reason for it. So little in human movement is straightforward and few rules exist—only guidelines. And those guidelines just keep getting expanded as we learn more.

Look again at the pitcher that we saw from figure 2.4 (below) and notice the lengthened tissues at the front of her right hip, how her lumbar and thoracic spine is extended, and the

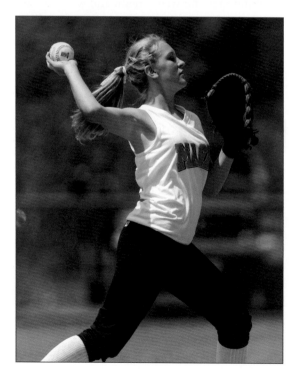

rotation between the pelvis and the rib cage. All of these areas of strain can help increase the force in the throw from her shoulder. But is each of those areas strained to the same degree?

Can you see how the anterior shoulder has opened quite a bit, her anterior abdominals have lengthened due to her spinal extension, but her right hip does not look as if it has extended much at all—the pelvis has anteriorly titled instead and further increased her spinal extension? In an overly-simplified analysis, we could suggest that her hip area is still in "zone 1," the abdominals have moved into "zone 2," and her right pectoralis major has created most of the leverage for the throw by going toward "zone 3."

Please keep in mind that the zones are arbitrary—they are a suggested vocabulary to link between the theory and the visual.

Working through chapters 4 to 7 will give plenty of opportunities to see how the body disperses and couples movement. We can then analyze which tissues should be lengthening in preparation for the return and which are less involved. Ideally, we would like to see each contributory soft tissue section move toward the same degree of strain. Any mismatches—areas that might be a "1" when others are a high "2," for example—would be reason to investigate.

Summary

Collagenous fascial tissues surround and support muscle fibers. The two tissue types, fascial tissue and muscle fiber, balance each other's strengths and weaknesses to create a system that is both efficient and strong, and capable of increasing its power output by using a countermovement strategy.

This chapter included an introduction to stress and strain, the elasticity of fascial tissue, and force-length and force-velocity relationships, all of which are worthy of much more detail than is possible to give here. Each dynamic is laid out in in most textbooks of biomechanics, but, although the books are useful sources for details, they rarely give enough context to inform the reader of the real-life implications. The intention of this chapter was to illustrate how each dynamic has implications for human movement, to provide the foundation on which you can build with further study if you wish.

Chapters 5 to 7 will show how movement patterns can influence strain distribution. When assessing quality of long-chain movement, we need to know the appropriate bone and joint reactions through the body and how much the corresponding tissues should strain. Using the definition of integration, each tissue should give an appropriate contribution—but what is "appropriate?"

During long-chain movements I want to see each tissue straining in concert with its neighbors. For example, if rectus abdominis is reaching into zone 3 during the cocking phase for a throw, then pectoralis major should also be reaching into zone 3. It would be inappropriate, or a mismatch, if rectus abdominis lengthened a lot but pectoralis major stayed short and in zone 1.

These zones are arbitrary divisions—the important point is to train our eyes to see consistent distribution of strain through the

whole system. That distribution of force will be contextual to the demands of the task. As we saw with the paper-throwing example, a short throw requires small degrees of strain in a few tissues. More powerful movements will recruit more tissues and require more strain through them to produce the necessary forces, and this is when tissue mechanics are particularly important to distribute the workload and prevent overuse injuries.

Reflection Questions

1. Why does the human body use a countermovement strategy?
2. What factors might influence the force used during such a movement?
3. Three length-related phases of myofascial units were outlined above. What are the differences between them, and when do we tend to operate within each range?
4. What is your understanding of *auxeticity*, and what are its implications for movement and strength?

Recommended Reading

Once upon a time fascia was relatively unknown in the world of bodywork and movement therapies; that has changed a lot in the last two decades. If you feel you have missed some of the detail on fascial tissues and want to know more, I recommend David Lesondak's excellent and easy-to-read introduction: *Fascia: What It Is and Why It Matters* (2nd ed., Handspring, 2022).

Much of the biomechanics in this chapter can be found in most introductory texts on the subject. The blending of fascial dynamics alongside it is less common and requires digging into expensive texts and less commonly accessed research articles, but a good introduction is also found in *Fascial Fitness* by Robert Schleip with Johanna Bayer (2nd ed., Lotus, 2021).

Anatomy Trains by Thomas W. Myers (Elsevier, 2020) also gives an introduction to the background of fascial tissues and the ways in which myofascial continuity might occur in the body.

Countermovement and the stretch-shortening cycle are well documented dynamics in strength and conditioning literature. Some of the leading names to research are Professor Anthony Blazevich (Edith Cowan University, Australia) and Professor Paavo Komi (who sadly died in 2018).

The following journal articles are also worth reading:

Ishikawa, M., J. Pakaslahti, and P. V. Komi, "Medial Gastrocnemius Muscle Behavior during Human Running and Walking," *Gait and Posture* 25, no. 3 (2007): 380–84.

Roberts, T. J., and E. Azizi, "Flexible Mechanisms: The Diverse Roles of Biological Springs in Vertebrate Movement," *Journal of Experimental Biology* 214 (2011): 353–61.

Van Wingerden, J. P., A. Vleeming, C. J. Snijders, and R. Stoeckart, "A Functional-Anatomical Approach to the Spine-Pelvis Mechanism: Interaction between the Biceps Femoris Muscle and the Sacrotuberous Ligament," *European Spine Journal* 2, no. 3 (1993): 140–44.

Wilke, Jan, Frieder Krause, Lutz Vogt, and Winfried Banzer, "What Is Evidence-Based about Myofascial Chains: A Systematic Review," *Archives of Physical Medicine and Rehabilitation* 97, no. 3 (2016): 454–61.

The first two papers cited above are relatively dense, the Wilke article is more easily accessible, but the paper I believe any dedicated reader should keep by their bedside is the Roberts and Azizi review article, as it gives an in-depth overview of the interactions between muscle and fascial tissues.

To further explore the concepts around force distribution through the body I also recommend reading any book by Stuart McGill. *Low Back Disorders: Evidence-Based Prevention and Rehabilitation* (Human Kinetics, 2015) is the more academic of his titles. *Back Mechanic* (self-pub., 2015) and *Ultimate Back Fitness and Performance* (5th ed., self-pub., 2004) both give solid overviews of his work and provide plenty of material for the serious therapist.

Orienting Ourselves

Maps are a way of organizing wonder.
—**Peter Steinhart**, ***Names on a Map***

Introduction

The last two chapters were about "why" we move the way we do. This chapter is about the "how"—not how we move, but how we can describe and communicate it. Finding a vocabulary for complex movement provides us with a map that empowers us to organize the complexity of what we see.

Any guide requires clear language for reference points, and, after critiquing anatomical position in chapter 1, I want to reestablish some of its credibility and show how it really helps our referencing system. Just as we saw the benefit of standardized measurements for length, weight, and volume, our ability to navigate ourselves around the word has developed through accepted conventions. There are many words that describe how we move through the world, and they help us know where we are and where we are going. Those words are useful, descriptive, and help us predict what will happen when we move.

Spending time practicing the vocabulary and language skills of anatomy will be time well spent. In my world of complementary therapy, there is often a resistance to the language of science. It can feel too pedantic, too difficult, and too, well, *sciencey*. Give it a chance, though, and it can become your most useful ally in the struggle to grasp the anatomy of movement.

Much of the reasoning behind the development of ideas, concepts, and vocabulary of anatomy has been diffused as it got handed down from teacher to teacher. By going back to see the original intention and the power behind it, we can regain clarity, and suddenly the world of movement opens up to us.

You may have been exposed to some of the ideas and words below—in fact, most anatomy books will show the planes of movement in the first few pages. But don't assume that I am about to repeat everything you have heard before. These next few pages will show you what has been missing in other texts and how you can use the concepts to rapidly expand your understanding.

To interpret, assess, or guide movement, it is essential that we share a vocabulary that is accurate and predictive.

The Real Secret to Understanding and Predicting Movement—Planes of Movement—but Don't Switch Off Just Yet

The virtue of maps, they show what can be done with limited space, they foresee that everything can happen therein.
—**José Saramago, *The Stone Raft***

Yes, the dreaded, boring planes! But, trust me, this will be less uncomfortable than flying transatlantic in cattle class—spend some time here and we'll have you sipping cocktails in the business section in no time. I know many people skim or even skip over the planes of movement—myself included, once upon a time—and consequently struggle to get the terminology straight in their heads.

Once that confusion has taken hold, we tend to ignore the planes of movement for the rest of our career. It is then easy to dismiss the planes as useless as we haven't needed them to get this far. However, as we often also complain that anatomy makes no sense of movement, there is a contradiction because the truth is that the tools were there all along, but we started by skipping over them. These tools are just the ones we need for a useful, descriptive, and predictive vocabulary of movement.

When teaching and discussing movement with other professionals, I often encounter resistance to the use of planes of movement

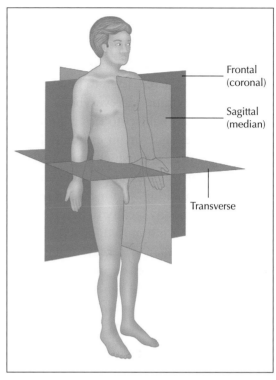

Figure 4.1. The planes of movement diagram is included in most textbooks and many people make the mistake of assuming that movement happens in one plane. Movement happens in each plane all the time, but most often a movement can be described by using the coordinate system of the planes.

(figure 4.1). I was once on a conference call discussing the anatomy of the pelvis and I asked a question about the frontal plane tilt of the pelvis during gait. A voice from the other end (this was pre-Zoom, and thankfully my face was not visible to anyone) said they did not believe in the planes of movement as the pelvis "just moves, and it moves in *spirals*."[1]

---

[1] For some reason "plane deniers" always want to place some kind of weird verbal emphasis on the spiral, and it is usually accompanied by some hand twirling. As I wasn't present for the hand twirling, I was treated to an even more exaggerated verbal "*spiii-rrr-alllls*."

Now, it is true that the pelvis moves, and it is true that the pelvis (and every other bone or joint) does not follow pure planar movement. Unchanging single-plane movement is restricted to physics textbooks; everything and everybody in the real world are subject to varying forces, uneven surfaces, and, in our examples here, irregular joint surfaces, which cause bones to twist and turn as they move. But simply saying that something "just moves in spirals" does not give me any facility to describe or measure how much it moved, how it moved differently today than yesterday, or how it differs from someone else's movement. Even the magical spiral would benefit from extra descriptors to let us know which direction it is traveling in, where it starts, where it ends, how tight or loose is the spiral, and how high and wide is its reach.

The use of *spirals* to describe movement creates the same problem as the *it could go anywhere* idea in tensegrity. Both statements might be true, but they don't provide us with any power to communicate the commonalities of movement inherent within our shared human anatomy. We need to befriend the language of anatomy, and, to do that, we have to see its value first.

> *Nature doesn't move in a straight line, and as part of nature, neither do we.*
> —**Gloria Steinem,**
> ***Revolution from Within***

The vocabulary exists to describe movement, not dictate it. This is a subtle but important point. Movement is complex and multidimensional, so we therefore need

multidimensional tools to describe it, and that is why the language of "planes" exists. The language is there only as a descriptive tool, one that we employ to illustrate how much movement occurs in certain directions, and the use of the three planar dimensions is a powerful tool that can describe complex spiral patterns (figure 4.2).

There are reasons for the confusion around the terminology of movement planes, as the terms are used in two ways. The first assumes precision and purity of the lines, and we see this in textbooks as cross-section images labeled *sagittal, frontal* (also known as the *coronal plane*), or *transverse plane* according to their orientation. Health-care reports use similar precision when asking for, or summarizing, the findings from imaging techniques (figure 4.3). When these images are coupled in our minds with the traditional planes of movement chart at the front of our anatomy texts, it creates another prejudice in

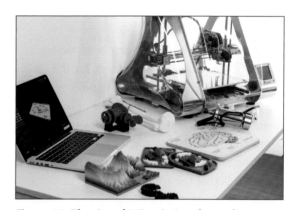

Figure 4.2. The rise of 3-D printing shows the power of using three coordinates. The movement of the continually moving print head is guided by 3-D plotting along the x, y, and z axes. Human movement can be just as beautiful and complex and can also be broken down into the same three axes—in anatomy we call them sagittal, frontal, and transverse.

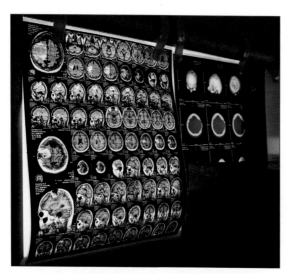

Figure 4.3. The planes are used to describe the orientation of the views we see in cross-sections and to position imaging technology to create views from appropriate angles.

our heads—the expectation of precise, linear movement.

There is a second way of using movement-plane terminology—one that enables our description and understanding of movement—and it is similar to the way we use the descriptors of joint movement. I have never heard anyone complain about the terms "flexion," "extension," "abduction," "adduction," or "rotation." We use the same terms to describe similar motions at very different joints. The knee and the elbow both flex and extend, but neither purely flexes—there is always some amount of rotation and abduction or adduction. While the amounts of other movement as we flex vary from joint to joint and person to person, we are all happy to call knee bending and elbow bending the same thing—"flexion."

If we can relax our intolerance of the use of the vocabulary of the planes of movement in the same way as we naturally do with the words we use to describe joint actions, a brave new world of descriptive power is instantly available to us. Viewing the planes not only as strict descriptors of a line (like in the MRI scans) but also in a manner akin to how we use compass points is far more useful to us in understanding the anatomy of movement. If I am being flown in an airplane, for example, I appreciate that the pilot will stay to a rigid, defined understanding of the cardinal points. If I meet her in the streets of New York and ask for directions along Fifth Avenue, however, I doubt she would stick to such a pedantic view, and nor would I need her to. We need to see and use the planes of movement in a similar, less pedantic and rigid, way.

I have difficulty orienting myself in space, and I'm probably one of the few people who gets lost in Manhattan.
—**Paul Auster**, *interview for Transatlantica*

For some reason, we are happy to orient ourselves in most grid-pattern cities according to, and using the language of, the points of the compass, even when the grid does not strictly follow the same lines. For example, the lines of Manhattan are oriented to the outline of the island, not to the cardinal points—points along Fifth Avenue are described as north or south, but the street actually runs northeast-southwest (figure 4.4).

If you have spent any time in New York City, you will know its citizens do not hold back on their criticism when there is something to complain about. Despite this, I have never

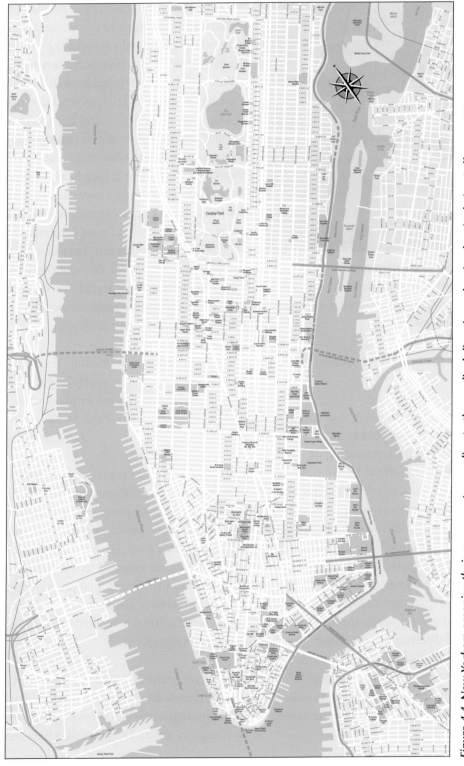

Figure 4.4. New Yorkers organize their movement according to the cardinal directions, despite the city being "off-center." Everyone accepts the looseness (or, perhaps, is unaware, or doesn't really care), and, to my knowledge, there has not been a campaign to reorient the city or to ban the use of the cardinal directions.

heard anyone shouting, yelling, or screaming that the streets and the compass points do not match.[2] There is a general acceptance that "close enough is good enough." The cardinal point system works, it is quick and easy, and it provides an efficient method for newcomers to the city.

This type of heuristic is exactly what we have been missing for describing movement.

We do not need a vocabulary that is perfectly accurate, nor must we assume that a vocabulary's intention is to *be* perfectly accurate, especially since being accurate for each and every one of us is an impossibility—there is too much variation in our anatomy and in our movement strategies for that degree of pedantry. As the purpose of this book is to help increase our understanding of movement, it is this "loose but useful" approach that we will take with the planes of movement.

Every movement can be mapped out using this system. The system helps us discuss the effects of movement in certain directions and how a movement has changed anatomical relationships, and facilitates prediction of what will happen in our bodies during a movement. I know that many people struggle with the terminology *sagittal*, *frontal*, and *transverse*, but that is because the terms are not used frequently enough to become second nature. With repetition, and a little help from some mnemonics, you will be fluent by the time you finish this text.

___

[2] If you ever do meet anyone with such a passion, suggest they move to Washington, DC, since its grid pattern *is* oriented to the cardinal points.

Planes of Motion, Bone Movement, and Joint Descriptors

Begin to look at maps with the narcotic tingle of possibility.
—**Rolf Potts**, *Vagabonding*

Much of the confusion around language is because we rarely define what is meant by each type of vocabulary. Clear descriptions of anatomy in movement require three levels of descriptor:

1. Words to describe the overall direction of movement—the planes of movement
2. Words to describe the reaction at each joint
3. Words to describe the motion of each individual bone.

By the time you finish this text, you will be fully armed with clear descriptors. At the moment you might not even be aware of the differences between them, or the reasons why you need them. I promise it will all become clear as you progress.

If you are a little nervous, don't be. You have already been using most of the words and following most of the conventions. It's possible that, because no one spelled out *why* they exist, you have simply lacked the context required to fully appreciate their significance.

We will explore anatomical reactions, or joint and bone motions (points 2 and 3 above), in later chapters.[3] This chapter will focus mainly on the planes of motion (point 1 above) and how they describe *movement direction*. We will reference anatomical reactions in each

___

[3] Points 2 and 3 will be further clarified in chapter 8.

of these directions, using active examples to help you embody the context of how all three descriptors fit together to fluently relate the anatomy of movement.

Understanding the differences between the descriptors is key to our accurate, useful, and predictive vocabulary. I know it might take some practice to settle in, and so we will revisit this from time to time throughout the text. For now, keep in mind that sagittal, frontal, and transverse motion can be used just like the compass points—we move forward and back, left and right, and we can turn left and right.

Getting Straight(ish) to the Point with the Sagittal Plane

The shortest distance between two points is often unbearable.
—Charles Bukowski

"Sagittal" has the same root as "Sagittarius," from the Latin for *arrow*. Although its etymology might go back earlier, adoption of the term into anatomy happened only in the twelfth century, with Italian translator Gerard of Cremona. Gerard used "sagittal" to describe the front-to-back suture along the top of the head, and, as you can see in figure 4.5b, he didn't intend it to indicate a perfectly straight line. Gerard was using the term "sagittal" in the same loose way we will—to indicate a general front-to-back direction.

The term "sagittal" orients us to the anterior-posterior direction, the direction in which we mostly flex and extend. Much of our

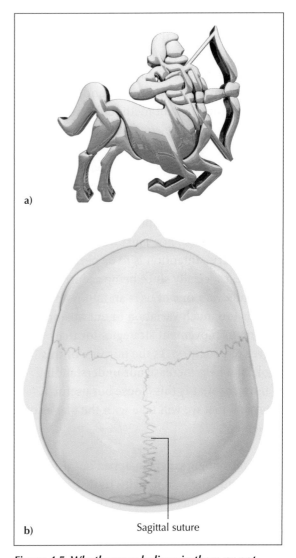

a)

b)   Sagittal suture

Figure 4.5. Whether you believe in them or not, most of us are familiar with the signs of the zodiac, and Sagittarius, the archer, is one of the most easily recognized (a). It shares part of its name with the wavy suture that runs front to back along the top of the head (b). That wavy line is an almost perfect representation of how an arrow flies once it leaves the bow—not in the perfectly straight line that we imagine (search YouTube for slo-mo arrows if you don't believe me).

locomotion occurs in this plane. It is common for others to point out that rotation also occurs during locomotion, but that is mixing up the levels of movement descriptors outlined above. "Sagittal" refers to the overall direction—getting from the Empire State Building to the MOMA along New York's Fifth Avenue (figure 4.4). The "rotations" are the responses in the bones and joints as we travel in that direction—our necessary sidesteps and arcs as we navigate traffic and other obstacles or landmarks along the way. As we progress forward, our bones will indeed tilt and rotate, and our joints will flex, extend, abduct, and adduct, and rotate. The differentiation is important—there is no contradiction in saying that sagittal plane movements are made of a series of bone and joint rotations. We would be wrong, though, if we were to say "we only rotate," or if we were to dismiss the sagittal description of an overall movement because we've confused ourselves with the rotational descriptions of the bones and joints involved.

Walking, running, skipping, and hopping are generally performed to take us forward—we need to get from A to B comfortably, safely, and, often, as quickly or efficiently as possible. Of course, we can do all those movements in different directions, but the most common movement is to step straight ahead with one foot in front of the other along the sagittal plane.

Our aim is to increase our ability to see and describe the interactions between movement and anatomy, and the best way to do this is to stand up and move. Position yourself comfortably for a quick and easy movement and anatomy experiment—stand with your feet on the floor, roughly hip-width apart, and at an angle that is comfortable for you. Now, swing your arms up and over your head, and then down toward your knees—swing back and forth a few times and feel what happens in your spine, hips, knees, and ankles (figure 4.6).

If you followed the instructions, you would probably have felt your spine flex and extend, your hips and knees flex and extend, and your ankles plantar flex and dorsiflex. The lesson is simple—movement that happens in the forward and backward (predominantly sagittal) plane causes the bones to tilt forward and backward, and causes the joints to flex and extend.

Full Exposure for the Frontal Plane

Many people struggle to remember the orientation of the frontal plane, and the method I used to imprint it was the fact that the "front" will always be visible in a true frontal plane motion. If we are looking at the front of the body, flexion and extension or any rotation will cause some of the body to disappear from view (figure 4.7). In this way, we could think that frontal plane movement keeps the body exposed.

We can employ a similarly simple exercise as we just used for sagittal movement to explore frontal plane movement. Starting in the same arms-up position and swinging our arms side to side over our heads (figure 4.8) will provoke side bending of the spine, *ad*duction and *ab*duction of the hips, and inversion and eversion at the ankle—all movements along the frontal plane.

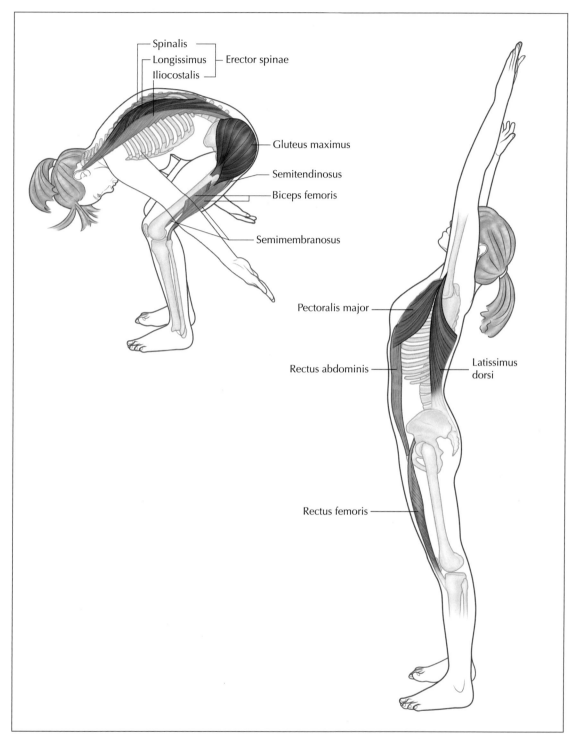

Figure 4.6. Standing in a comfortable neutral, bring your arms overhead and then swing them forward and down, up and back, and repeat.

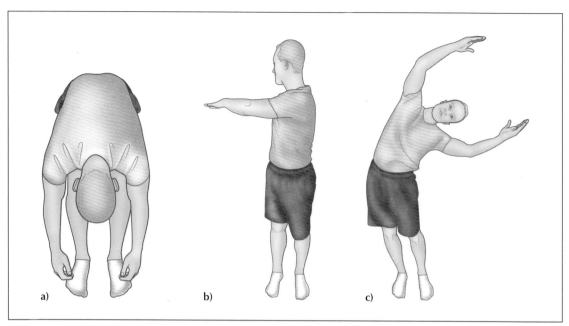

Figure 4.7. Movement in the (a) sagittal (flexion/extension) and (b) transverse planes (rotation) will take some parts of the body out of sight when viewed from the front. (c) Frontal plane movement (side flexion, adduction and abduction, inversion and eversion) keeps it all in sight. It is important to remember that this is only an aide-mémoire. Frontal plane movement will be combined with movements in the other planes, and therefore parts will constantly come and go from view during real-life movement.

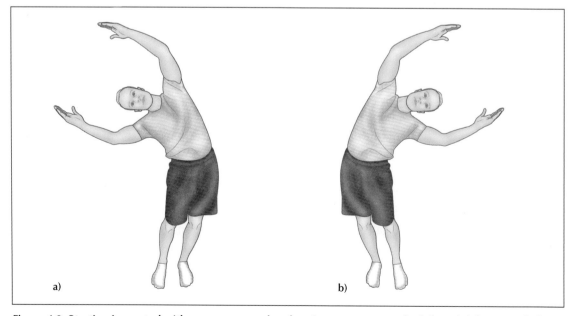

Figure 4.8. Starting in neutral with your arms overhead, swing your arms to the left and right. Frontal plane motion causes the bones to tilt left and right, and the joints to abduct, adduct, invert, evert, and side flex.

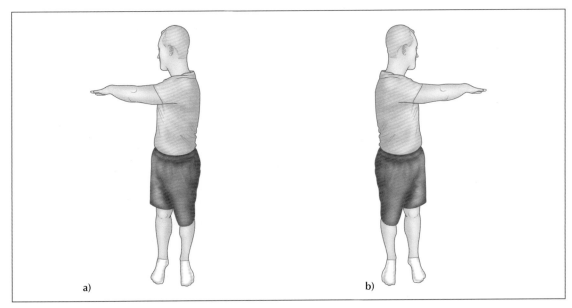

a)   b)

Figure 4.9. Swinging your arms left to right in the transverse plane causes a series of rotations through the body.

Finally, the Turn of the Transverse Plane

> *The song of the curved line is called happiness.*
> —**René Crevel,** *My Body and I*

Few people struggle to remember the transverse plane—it is all about rotation and is omnipresent in every movement we make.

To experience the reaction in the transverse plane, bring your arms straight out in front of you and swing them left to right (figure 4.9). It should be no surprise that transverse plane movement causes rotations through the body—in the spine and hips, in this case. You may also feel your feet adapt by alternately pronating and supinating as you swing from one side to the other.

Although it is possible to have anatomical variations that create different responses, most of us will have similar reactions to these movements if we:

1. Make the arm movements large enough and with enough momentum
2. Allow the body to respond naturally and do not try to prevent the reaction travel-through: For example, many movement teachers will "stabilize the pelvis" during the movement, which inhibits the lower body from reacting and limits its response to the upper body's movement. Similarly, an injury—old or new—could prevent you from letting the reaction happen.[4]
3. Make sure your environment allows the natural response: If you did the exercise sitting on a chair, the contact with the

---

[4] Is this starting to sound like interesting information that you might like to be able to spot when a client presents to you?

chair would inhibit the reaction into the lower body. If you are wearing supportive, tight shoes or orthotics, you also might not feel the feet reacting in the same way.

Confidence Builder—the Dummy's Guide to Planes and Movement

Words play an enormous part in our lives and are therefore deserving of the closest study.

—**Aldous Huxley,** *Words and Their Meanings*

Now that you've felt for yourself all the movements in the different planes, and all the reactions in the joints involved, you can use the following summary as a handy, albeit simplified, aide-mémoire. Each of these statements has some truth, and, while they are all open to debate, they will help us to organize and remember the relationships between movement and joint reactions:

- **Sagittal plane movement** is related to **joint flexion** and **extension**.
- **Frontal plane movement** is related to **joint abduction** and **adduction**, and **ankle (subtalar joint) inversion** and **eversion**, and **spinal (joint) side flexion**.
- **Transverse plane movement** is related to **joint rotation pronation, and supination of the feet**.

| Coupled Motions

Understanding the preceding three simple relationships between movement direction and joint reactions will boost your ability to see what is happening during movement. But remember—no joint ever moves in a single plane.

Joint descriptors, such as flexion, extension, abduction and adduction, are just a shorthand method for describing the general reaction at the joint. Remember, elbow flexion is not the same movement as knee flexion—the arrangement of bone shapes and soft tissues tends to cause the bones to tilt and rotate as they move. Bones do not swivel on fixed hinges, they move in each plane during any movement, and some bones will move more in certain directions than others.

If you have studied anatomy to some degree, you will know that each joint has characteristic motions. Joints never purely flex, abduct, or rotate—there is always some combination of these, and the combination is predictable. These so-called *coupled motions*, often cited in the spine as Fryette's laws, or the "screw-home mechanism" of the knee, should take place at each joint and with each motion.

All I know is what I have words for.
—**Ludwig Wittgenstein,** *Tractatus Logico-Philosophicus*

We can learn about motion coupling at different levels—the first is at joint level, which is how it is most often discussed. Coupled motion at a joint is used to describe the three-dimensionality of a bone's movement as it moves through its joint. For example, the tibia will rotate as the knee flexes and extends. This is due to the architecture of the joint and the bones involved.

The second way in which we can think of coupling is the linkage between different areas of the body. For example, the naturally limited ranges of motion in the knees cause an overall movement to travel further below the knees and into the ankles and feet—in our examples above, frontal and transverse plane movement of the upper body was *coupled* from the pelvis to the feet because of the lack of rotation, abduction, and adduction available at the knee. This is why you felt your ankles evert and invert, and your feet pronate and supinate— had the knees been capable of side flexion and/ or rotation, everything below the knees would have remained still.

Movements in certain directions communicate through our bodies in reasonably predictable patterns. In our exercises above, the swing of the arms in each direction caused the joints to react in each plane—but not every joint contributed in the same way in each direction. Some joints move more easily in certain directions than others, as we saw with the knee's ability to flex and extend and its limitations in rotation, adduction, and abduction.

Learning the coupled motions of the individual joint helps one know what is likely to happen in that joint. For example, when someone makes a sagittal plane movement, the knee should flex and extend and the bones in the knee joint should also rotate, according to the screw-home mechanism. There are no contradictions here, and this is the beauty of being able to separate out the three levels of motion descriptor as described above. It is through specificity that we become fluent. (A reminder—those three levels are: (1) the overall movement direction, (2) the joint reaction, and (3) the direction of movement of each bone.)

Many resources are available if you'd like to learn the coupled motions of individual joints.[5] This text will focus on how the human body couples motion through its entire tensegral body. We will explore coupling between tissues throughout the text, building up the picture of how and why coupling happens and what it means for us in practice.

"Normal Movement" and Movement Restrictions

I don't see normal movement—I see things in very complicated shots.
—**Penelope Cruz,** *interview for Interview magazine*

The natural lack of movement in one or two planes in a joint is not necessarily a bad thing—indeed, it is essential in many cases— and we should certainly not try to increase ranges of motion that should not be there. If a joint's architecture limits its contribution in the direction we move, the momentum of the movement of one bone will pass through the joint to the next bone to create a coupling action.

To experience the effect of joint contributions and coupling in long-chain movement, stand again, and look at your right hand as you turn all the way to your right (figure 4.10a). Try to reach around as far as you comfortably can without either repositioning your feet or causing

---

[5] We do not have space here to investigate coupled motion for every joint. Resources for such a pursuit are suggested at the end of the chapter.

discomfort. Allow your body to react naturally to the movement and take note of:

1. The distance that you turned: We will call this your overall *range of movement*.
2. The reaction in your left foot: Did it pronate?

Next, repeat the same movement, but this time stop your left foot from pronating (figure 4.10b).

What happened to your overall range of movement when you restricted the pronation of the left foot? Could you reach as far? Now repeat the movement again without pronating your left foot and try to achieve the same overall range as the first movement (figure 4.10c). Where do you notice yourself compensating for the loss of range of motion in the foot?

To compensate for reduced *range of movement* due to a restricted *range of motion* at an individual joint, most people will increase a *range of motion* somewhere else through the kinetic chain.

Differentiating between range of movement and a range of motion is extremely useful. We operate in the real world with ranges of movement, which are the accumulation of motions from a chain of joints.

During functional, real-life movement our system does not organize itself on a joint-by-joint basis, it just wants to get the job done. The body recruits some movement from a sequence of joints and tissues, and if one or two don't give enough, the body will ask for more movement from somewhere else, and there will be an unequal or inappropriate

distribution of strain. We saw this uneven distribution in the analysis of the softball pitcher in the previous chapter.

While everyone will have a slightly different reaction during the exercise in figure 4.10, the possibilities are that you may have felt some extra strain at the front of the right shoulder, or compression at the back, or perhaps you experienced something in your ribs or spine, a torsion through your pelvis, or a twist of your knee.

Each of these reactions is normal, as we tend to overuse one (or more) area(s) to compensate for a loss of range in another (or others). There is value in understanding this because there is a potential cost to any localized overreach. That cost may be different for each of us, so we should avoid applying sweeping assumptions or expectant catastrophizing, which often invoke generic treatment protocols. The truth is that, until we observe and experiment, we do not know what will happen in those areas that move more than they "should"—and we shouldn't even use the word "should!" There is a delicate line we must tread, as we develop our movement vocabulary, in our use of the term "normal," since "normal" automatically assumes deviations from it to be "abnormal."

What we will focus on for the rest of this text is the *usual*, the *common*, or the *most likely* reactions through the body in response to movement. As I have said before, this book is designed to build the vocabulary and understanding of movement to give us tools for assessing, directing, and perhaps suggesting alternative strategies. We will leave what is "correct," "best," "harmful,"

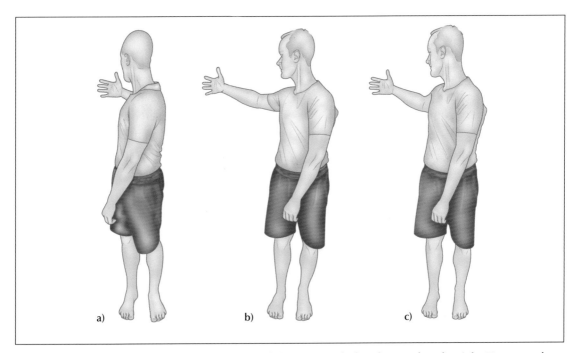

a) b) c)

Figure 4.10. (a) Feel your body's reactions as you follow your right hand around to the right. Try to reach as far as is comfortable without shifting your feet. Notice how far you reach and then return to neutral. (b) Either place something under your left foot or imagine something being there to stop it from pronating. (c) Repeat the same movement without letting your left foot pronate. Try to reach the same point as before without giving yourself an injury.

A relatively normal reaction is for the rotation to pass through the whole body as the arm reaches back. The spine and pelvis turn, and the right foot supinates while the left pronates. Restricting motion of the left foot reduces the whole range of movement (b). Note how the pelvis remains relatively neutral in (b) and (c), but the loss of pronation is compensated for by increased rotation of the trunk in (c).

or "dangerous" to those who prefer to proselytize and scaremonger on social media. The only expert in the room is the owner of their own body and the reference point for all interventions should be themselves.

That is not to say that the role of any therapist or movement teacher is passive or redundant. A therapist's role is to facilitate a client's exploration, discuss reasons why certain patterns may have developed, help search for other movement strategies if they are needed, and encourage, reassure, support, and guide anyone in pain or discomfort.

The subject of pain is complex, and our understanding of it has greatly improved over the last decade. While this text will not pretend to answer all the biomechanical issues that may or may not be at fault, we can lay out the common movement reactions during long-chain movement and, thereby, assist your recognition of when an area is not contributing appropriately. Addressing those "quiet" areas, like the lack of pronation in the left foot during the exercise above, can be very productive for the client, who—working with their therapist or alone—may find ways to bring some respite to mechanically overstrained areas.

Bringing the Movement and Anatomy Together

The technicalities matter a lot, but the unifying vision matters more.
—**Ted Nelson,** *Computer Lib/Dream Machines*

There is much that we can learn from the four introductory exercises above (figures 4.6 and 4.8–4.10). The first and perhaps most important is that movement direction creates reasonably predictable reactions in our bodies (outlined above in the "Confidence Builder"). Work through this book and you will have the ability to predict and describe each of those reactions.

You will be able to predict and describe anatomical reactions to movement because the architecture of the joints determines much of their response to motion. For example, as we have already seen, the knee joints are "designed" with a large range of flexion and extension but very little rotation or *ad/ab*duction.

The predictions work in both directions. We know sagittal plane movement is likely to use knee flexion/extension, which means that we know that knee flexion/extension can be used for sagittal plane movement. Depending on whether the knees are reacting (as in the exercises above) or acting to create a movement (such as a squat), this can be invaluable information when seeking to understand (and possibly change) a person's movement.

Similarly, joint architecture can allow the joint to move in the direction of the overall movement, or it can prevent the joint from contributing, depending on its "design." Continuing with the knees as an example, the first movement, in the sagittal plane, created knee flexion and extension. Relatively little happened in the knee joints during the second and third frontal and transverse plane movements (some movement does happen, but it is slight). The reduced movement available in the knee joint for frontal and transverse plane movements led to more movement in the ankle joints and feet via coupled motion.

Summary

There are many important vocabulary tools in this chapter—planes; movement and motion; the differentiation between long-chain movement, joint motion, and bone motion; range of movement and range of motion; and coupled motions, both within joints (Fryette's laws and the screw-home mechanism) and between joints (the communication of motion from one bone to others). Don't expect to be fluent with them just yet—the details are here for you to review and come back to, but do work through the questions below and we will come back to the principles of planes, movement, motion, and coupling with each chapter as you progress through the book.

Further Reading

There are many other resources available to explore the links between anatomy and movement. Although each of them is worthy of investigation, keep in mind that few authors are attentive to the important differences between describing overall movement, the motions at joints, and the motion of bones. Some of the authors I recommend are:

Joanne Elphinston
Todd Hargrove
Jules Mitchell
Diane Lee
Robert Schleip and his approach to "fascial fitness"

If you wish to venture into more detail on the coupled motions of joints, please see the excellent *Physiology of the Joints* by I. A. Kapandji (3 vols., 7th ed., Handspring, 2019), and Serge Gracovetsky's fascinating *The Spinal Engine* (Springer-Verlag, 1988).

Reflection Questions

Life doesn't move in straight lines, and neighter does a good conversation.
    —**Margaret J. Wheatley,**
    Turning to One Another

1. Can you name the three planes of movement?
2. What do you understand by each of the names?
3. Generally, how do the joints react when performing movements in each plane?
4. What do you understand by the differentiation between "range of movement" and "range of motion"?
5. There are two ways in which motion is "coupled" through the body—can you explain them?
6. What are the possible implications to strain distribution if one joint has a reduced range of motion? Can you think of examples in your own body during certain movements?

Stepping Forward

Where Are We Starting From?

Pursued by our origins … we all are.
—**Emil M. Cioran,** *History and Utopia*

Despite all mammals having the same general skeletal plan, human posture and locomotion are unique. Our upright stance developed through a few small but important changes. The overall body pattern of vertebrates has not altered much in terms of the presence and position of bones and their joints—we can recognize and name most of the crocodile bones without any knowledge of reptilian anatomy (figure 5.1; see also figure 2.1). What have changed are the lengths and sizes of many of the bones and, importantly, the alignment of the joints.

An early adaptation of the mammalian skeleton was medial rotation at the hip joints (figure 5.2),

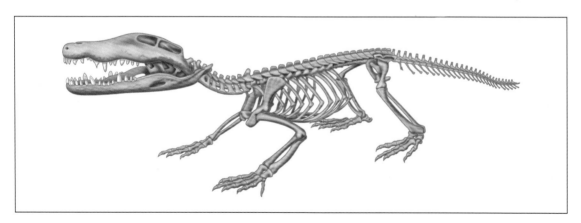

Figure 5.1. There is a general consistency to the vertebrate body plan. Each species has more or less the same bones in the same places, but they differ in size, shape, and orientation. It is those differences that create variation in locomotor patterns. For example, each bone of the lower limb of the crocodile is similar to ours but we can see the knee joint faces outward rather than straight ahead.

which brought the knee joint toward the front of the body rather than out to the side. This reorientation is something our human ancestors took advantage of—the new joint alignments and ranges were part of the development of our upright stance, especially once lumbar extension had increased. Developing a lumbar lordosis was critical to standing and walking comfortably with our head directly above our feet. The efficiency of our relatively straight-legged gait was enhanced by changes at the feet and ankles. Adduction of the big toe, developing a domed foot, and torsion through the tibia all brought the toe, ankle, knee, and lumbar spinal joints into a generally sagittal plane alignment.

Although much of our movement might be rotational, it has been the realignment

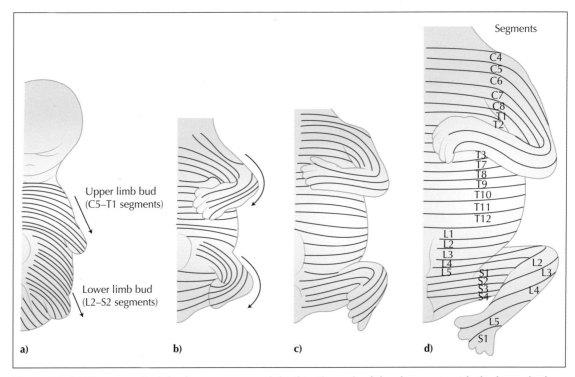

Figure 5.2. (a) The upper limb buds appear around the fourth week of development, with the lower limb buds a week later. (b and c) Over the next two to three weeks, the distal ends flatten to form hand- and footlike paddles as the proximal portions of the upper limb torsion laterally and the lower limb torsions medially. (d) Below the knee, the lower limb continues to twist to bring the great toe to the medial aspect. The lines indicate the spinal segmentation of innervation to the skin (each segment known as a dermatome), presented here for visual clarity of the torsions that occur during development. The in utero rotation of the lower limb reorients the knee, talar, and toe joints close to the sagittal plane and causes the ligaments of the hip to twist around the front of the hip. The torsion of the ligaments helps them limit extension and protect the integrity of the hip joint.

into the sagittal plane of some major joints that has allowed us to stand and walk with straight legs. However, our upright stance brings us toward the end of range of most of the major joints—the patella, the twisted ligaments around the front of the hip joint, and the lumbar facets will all limit any further movement into extension. While the changes have helped produce an efficient posture, they have also placed some limits on how we move, as we now have much greater potential for movement into flexion than into extension because we are starting from an extended position.

The last few years have seen a number of fear-based social media campaigns warning us of the various dangers of "text-neck" and "sitting—the new smoking." These inflammatory and overstretched comments are trying to pathologize the flexion that is built into our vertebral anatomy, when the truth is we have been bending forward to perform tasks for many millions of years. We should also appreciate that we live close to the natural limits of extension in our bodies and cannot go much further into extension. However, those few degrees of extension that we can go into are important to us, especially when we need a few extra units of force.

As we saw earlier, we use countermovements (usually into extension) to prepare for almost every action that requires extra force. The preparatory movement is rarely limited to a single joint—it is the accumulated range of movement through a series of tissues that gives more leverage. When beginning a movement from anatomical neutral, it is only the shallow-socketed glenohumeral joint that

has much extension available. But even though the rest of the upper body's joints give just a few degrees, they still add up to something useful, especially as they recruit their related soft tissues into the overall movement. This is the difference between the *range of motion* of individual joints and the *range of movement* of our overall system—the range of movement is the accumulation of the ranges of motion, and the therapist needs to look for and assess both.

Before looking for movement through an area, I recommend seeing where the joints are starting from—are they already extended, or is the person starting from a flexed position? I use postural assessment less to focus on the significance of quiet standing and more to ask: "When this person moves, where are their joints starting movement from?" To appreciate the range of motion through any joint, I must see where the movement started from—a more interesting and potentially important question to ask when looking at posture.

Exploring Our Limits

The greatest discoveries all start with the question "Why?"

—**Robert Ballard**

Each of the movements illustrated below could be adapted as exercises, stretches, general mobilizations … as anything you want, really. The illustrations are here to help us build pattern recognition of what happens during relatively simple movements, so we start to recognize what happens in more complex ones.

One of the first movements we explored in chapter 4 was the simple forward and back bilateral arm swing to illustrate how our major joints are aligned close to the sagittal plane (figure 4.6). The metatarsophalangeal (MTP) joints, the talar joint, the knee joint, and the overall range of the spinal facets are biased toward flexion and extension, and contribute to our gait pattern. Our long, straight-legged stride relies on our ability to extend through these joints, and the alignment of the lower limb helps bring strain to the front of the hip joint.

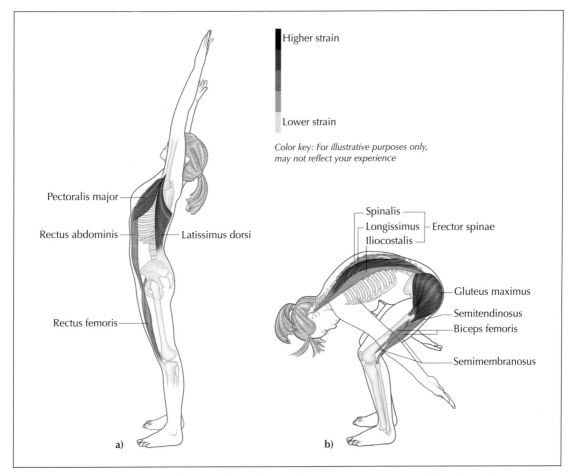

Figure 5.3. (a) Bringing both hands up and over the shoulders can bring us toward the limits of our extension possibilities. The large shoulder movement untwists the fibers of the pectoralis major and latissimus dorsi, which strain to support the humerus in its shallow socket. The rectus abdominis strains to support spinal extension, which—although the range is small between any pair of vertebrae—is cumulatively quite large through the entire spine. Hip extension is limited by the already-twisted ligaments supporting the joint capsule, and knee extension is prevented by the patella. (b) In contrast to the ligamentous and bony limitations for extension, joint flexions at the knee, hip, elbow (not shown), and spine are often limited by tissue approximation. The increased range of flexion lets us protect our vulnerable ventral tissues.

We saw earlier how the hip joint twists in utero to bring the dorsal surface of the lower limb to the front, winding up the ligaments at the front of the hip (figure 5.2). The wrap-around nature of these ligaments allows them to unwind as we flex the hip joint but draw tighter as we extend and limit our hip extension to 12°–15°. We can see the difference between our flexion and extension ranges in figure 5.3. Our bodies naturally fold into flexion for protection (figure 5.3b), but extension, used for preparation during many ballistic movements, is limited by several anatomical features (figure 5.3a).

Going Forward to Go Back

Life can only be understood backwards; but it must be lived forwards.
—**Søren Kierkegaard, *Journals*, 1843**

We have already discussed the principles of elastic loading and the stretch-shortening cycle as efficient movement strategies, and we have seen how most of our movements, especially when we want to create more power, start by going in the opposite direction from the intended, ultimate direction. But there are other dynamics that determine overall movement patterns as well. Both movements in figure 5.3 finish with the ankle in dorsiflexion, even though the first movement was into extension and the second into flexion.

There are a number of reasons why we tend to prefer moving into dorsiflexion rather than plantar flexion. The first is because of our extended knee position when standing—to go into plantar flexion would require

the knee to extend, but it can't go into any further extension because the patella blocks the movement. Knee flexion and ankle dorsiflexion are quite closely coupled—try dorsiflexing your ankles without flexing your knees; then try flexing your knees without dorsiflexing your ankles. The movements can be done, but it is quite unstable and hard work.

The second main reason for our dorsiflexion bias is because we are starting from a relatively "plantar flexed" position. Other plantigrade species tend to carry their body weight forward of their feet owing to their dorsiflexed ankle, flexed knees, and flexed hips (figure 5.1).[1] Our upright stance has brought our tibia into a more vertical position, which reduces the workload on the calf muscles. However, we feel more stable if we bring our body weight forward over our feet during movement—an action that uses dorsiflexion.

In some traditions dorsiflexion is referred to as "extension" and plantar flexion as "flexion." This is due to the rotation of the lower limb in utero (figure 5.2). The rotation brought our major joints into a general alignment with the sagittal plane, and it reversed the flexion/extension direction in the lower limb. The talar joint is therefore the one joint in our body that flexed rather than extended to help us stand upright. (We will explore the reversal of the lower limb further below.)

The natural architecture of the rear foot and ankle, with our center of gravity arranged vertically above it, means we cannot move

---

[1]*Plantigrade* is the technical term for animals that walk on the whole of the foot rather than on their toes. Those that walk on their toes are termed *digitigrade*.

our body weight back very far. We have a few anatomical elements that help us—an extended heel, and a posteriorly projecting ischial tuberosity (figure 5.4)—but they are small. Stability is difficult for us to achieve during backward movement. Not only can we not extend our knees back further, but our heels do not have the length to support us much beyond the axis of the talar joint. Coming forward into joint flexions lets us keep our center of gravity over our feet—the spine, hips, and ankles bend forward, while the knee uses its larger range into flexion to keep our body weight under control.

We also use a natural pattern of folding into flexion to help decelerate and control impact forces. Whether we jump from a height or have to navigate repeated ground reaction forces during a run, our natural, joint-determined, and soft-tissue-friendly strategy is to dorsiflex the ankles and flex the knees and hips. If we are running, those three joints may be adequate to recruit enough soft tissue to absorb the impact forces, but landing from a height will probably also draw the spine into flexion. It is a simple formula—the more force involved, the more tissue must be recruited. This formula is true in reverse as well—whether we are absorbing forces or trying to create extra power for a jump, the more height that is involved, the more bend in the joints we are likely to use.

The relationship between joint architecture and soft tissue alignment works in both directions. By contracting concentrically, muscles will create movement through the joints—when dealing with impact, the forces involved will be sent via the joints into the soft tissues, to allow them to react and control the forces by adjusting their length and tension before any damage is done (hopefully).

The arrangement of muscles around the joints is directly related to our natural movement tendencies. It seems almost too obvious to say, but I think we sometimes fail to appreciate the interrelationship between joint range, soft-tissue groupings, and our movement potentials. These three dynamics must correlate if we are to move successfully. There is no point, and it would be unstable and dangerous, to have a joint movement without the muscle to control it. Although the performers of Cirque du Soleil might make it look as if any movement is possible, most of us cannot move our body in directions that defy the natural lumps, bumps, and grooves of our joints, or the limitations of our soft tissues.

Joint movement, direction, and control of movement all intertwine, and we especially see that in the alternating strengths of muscular arrangement in the lower limb. As we tend to use dorsiflexion to absorb and produce force, most of the muscles below the knee joint are plantar flexors, including the very strong soleus (figure 5.5).[2] We then see something similar at the front of the thigh, with the vast bulk of the quadriceps available to decelerate knee flexion. Finally, at the top of the lower limb we then switch to the back of the body again to find the famously strong gluteal muscles to control hip flexion.

---

[2]Remember, the term "leg" refers only to the lower portion of the lower limb—the bit below the knee.

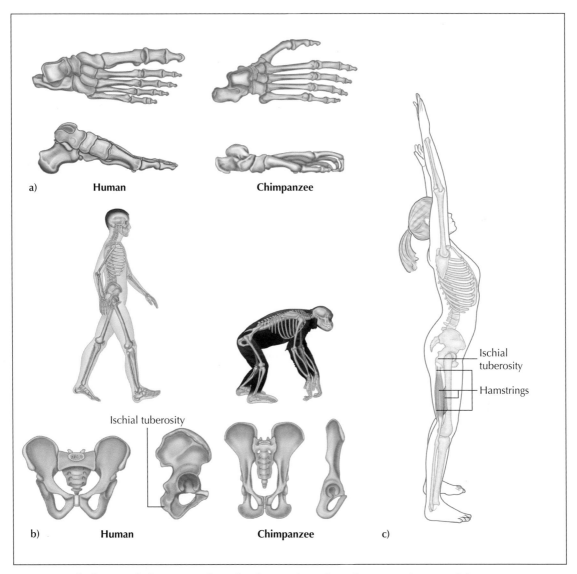

Figure 5.4. The human skeleton contains a few interesting adaptations to assist an upright stance. The human calcaneus projects further posteriorly, and as the human heel bears more weight than the chimpanzee heel our calcaneus needs to be more robust (a). There are many differences between the human and chimpanzee pelves. One that is rarely discussed in the general literature is the posterior projection of the human ischial tuberosity. When pitched forward (b), the chimpanzee can use the leverage provided by the inferior projection of the ischial ramus, but that advantage is lost when the chimpanzee stands upright. When compared side to side, we can see the hamstring attachment in the human pelvis extends further backward than that of the chimpanzee (c). Could that be one reason why some people anteriorly tilt their pelvis when performing certain movements? The anterior tilt increases the angle between the tibia and the ischium and provides the hamstrings muscles more potential to help control the pelvis. If this is the case, the anterior tilt is not a flaw but may be a compensation for weakness in another area, such as the abdominals.

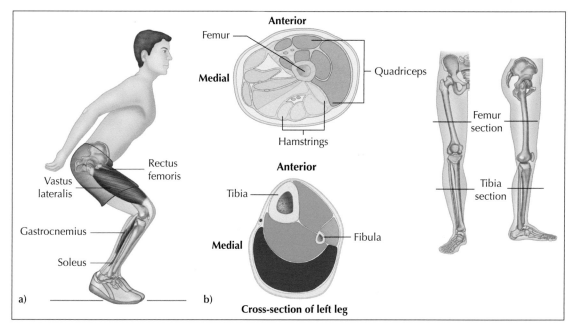

Figure 5.5. (a) Our natural way to control high forces through the lower limb is to dorsiflex the ankles, flex the knees and hips, and flex the spine. The reverse motions are used for recovery and to jump or propel forward when running or hopping. Both actions—the absorption of force through the flexions, and the production of force through extensions—use the same alternating pattern of major muscle groups.
(b) The soft tissues must have the power and strength to deal with high levels of force, and one solution is to allocate more muscle bulk for these roles. The quadriceps are significantly larger and stronger than the hamstrings; at the ankle, the plantar flexors outnumber and outpower the dorsiflexors; likewise at the hip with the gluteals and the hip flexors.

Myofascial Continuities—Fact or Fiction, Useful or Distraction?

Continuity is how you build a physique.
—**Frank Zane**

The long lines of stretch or strain through the front and back of the body during sagittal movements appear to overlap with the superficial front line and back lines from Myers's anatomy trains model (figure 5.6). As we have seen earlier, there is limited evidence to support the idea of the superficial front line as a myofascial continuity.

However, the vertical tissues on the front of the body (figure 5.3a) do not have to be directly continuous to help create or control movement. If the muscle fibers of different muscles are aligned in the direction bones are moving, the fibers will directly influence the movement with or without continuity between the myofascial units.

The lack of myofascial continuity becomes less significant if we focus not on the anatomy but on the movement. Look at the line of strain through the front of the body as the arms are taken back in figure 5.3a—there is a

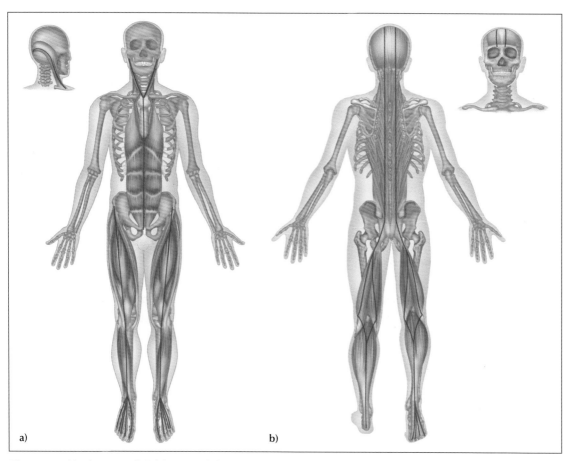

Figure 5.6. (a) The superficial front and (b) superficial back lines, according to Myers.

continuous line of strain that matches the *idea* of the superficial front line (SFL), if not the reality. The tissues listed as part of the SFL—the sternocleidomastoid, sternalis, rectus abdominis, quadriceps (especially the rectus femoris in this example), and the anterior compartment of the leg—will all have some degree of strain in them, although comparatively more in the rectus femoris and rectus abdominis.

A second consideration is that tissues do not have to be directly myofascially continuous to transfer force between them. As mentioned in chapter 2, support for this idea comes from research performed by Dutch anatomist Andry

Vleeming when he and his group showed the sacrotuberous ligament was tensioned by straining the biceps femoris regardless of the degree of fascial connection between the two structures.

In the case of the SFL, the two rectus muscles are the main cause for concern in terms of continuity—they are not directly continuous. However, they are connected through the pelvis, and, just like Vleeming's "unconnected" biceps femoris and sacrotuberous ligament, this bony connection indicates communication of force through the skeleton. But isn't that kind of true for everything through the whole body? The body is continuous with itself, so what is all the fuss about?

Well, the fuss is because knowing how the body communicates forces can be useful, so that we can adjust movements or have better interpretations of what is going on by understanding tissue directions and continuity. Over the last couple of decades, our focus has moved away from bones and joints and toward myofascia, especially with the idea of continuity. However, just as the fascia is continuous through the body, so is everything else, and it all needs to be seen in context.

We cannot separate the abilities of the soft tissues from the alignments of the joints, and, when it comes to movement, the thing that controls them all will be the all-pervasive nervous system. While it may be tempting to see the movements in this book as expressions of myofascial continuities, they are much better seen as the orchestration of joints, soft tissues, and motor control, along with the glides and slides of the many visceral tissues that also must adapt to allow movement to happen.

One of the many issues with focusing on myofascial continuities is that this tends to limit our attention to that particular line of tissue, which can then undermine the importance of tissues at other depths. Although it is common to now challenge the idea of "layers" in the body because of the body's accepted continuity, the concept of layers is still useful—just as we saw with the concept of levers and leverage earlier.[3] It is

therefore important that we use the *idea* of lines without getting lost in their detail. We should talk about not only the rectus femoris or abdominis but everything that is in front of the spine and in front of the hips.

Seeing, thinking about, and spending time learning each line creates a focusing dynamic, and we may start to lose sight of the many other important elements that contribute to movement.

For example, in the extension pattern of figure 5.4c:

- There is a change in the center of gravity over the feet as the pelvis moves forward.
- The ankle is dorsiflexed, whereas plantar flexion would be a consistent strain of the SFL.
- The arms and shoulders—not part of the SFL—are involved.
- Most importantly, to achieve extension, the spine and everything between it and the skin must contribute to the movement.

The focus should also move beyond the musculoskeletal tissues to recognize the many roles of the nervous system and how it might organize a movement based on the client's history of sports, injuries and trauma, expectation, or interpretation of what the movement should look like. Rather than focusing on training the tissues, we should consider training movement patterns and creating a safe space for the client and their nervous system.

---

[3]The significance of anatomical layering is revisited in chapter 6.

The Ventral Line

Another controversial anatomy train is the so-called "deep front line," which has not been fully or independently researched for credibility (figure 5.7). I would like to include a discussion of it here, as it illustrates several points about human movement, our evolutionary past, and how the two combine.

The first things to notice about the deep front line is that it is not always particularly *deep*, nor does it follow the *front* of the body. Myers claims the myofascial tissues are continuous from the front of the jaw to the back of leg and into the soles of the feet; the line passes through the trunk and its viscera, and into the adductors via the pelvic floor and deep hip flexors. The jaw, throat, and adductor muscles are not particularly deep, and the lower

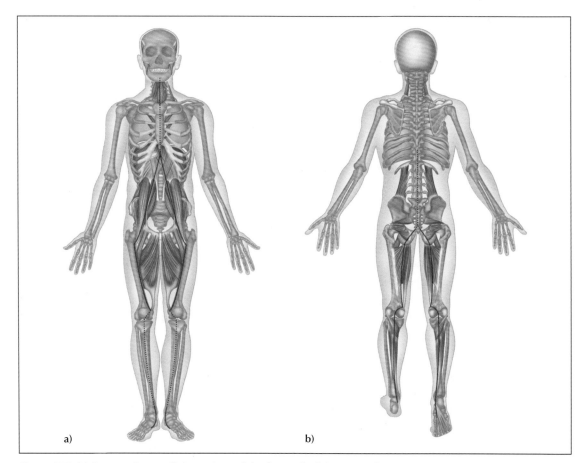

a)   b)

Figure 5.7. (a) Due to the medial rotation of the lower limb in utero (figure 5.2), Myers's proposed deep front line actually follows the body's ventral tissue. Composed of predominantly flexor muscles, this line is then tensioned by and helps control extension, which happens at a series of joints through the body in many everyday human movements. (b) Taking a step forward leaves one foot behind and the joints in that trailing limb create an almost perfect strain through the ventral tissues.

portion of Myers's deep *front* line uses the muscles of the deep *posterior* compartment to join the thigh to the foot.

The one thing all these tissues have in common is their position on our *ventral* surface (see below). They are all flexor-related tissues and therefore tensioned as we move into extension. Although it is still to be established if any of this line can communicate strain along it, we can still use the image of the line to highlight interrelated events that happen during many of our most common movements.

Notice the consistency of the actions of the muscles of the ventral line (psoas, iliacus, anterior adductors, tibialis posterior, and flexors hallucis and digitorum longus)—they are all flexors. Each of them is contributing to control the movement, and the overall movement is coordinated along and through this richly innervated series of tissues. It makes perfect sense that these ventral tissues would be connected and capable of transferring force. However, that is far from proven and remains conjecture, based on a few dissections and assumptions drawn from our embryology.

Front, Back, Ventral, or Dorsal?

I go back so far I'm in front of me.
—**Paul McCartney,**
"The World Tonight"

Whether we consider the myofascial tissue as continuous or not, the line of strain travels through the body in reasonably consistent vectors. For example, a lunge-type position (figure 5.8) mimics the step that we saw in figure 5.7b, and we can use the image of myofascia that create vertical forces along the front of the body—the rectus abdominis, rectus femoris—and the plantar flexors at the back of the calf to show the strain pattern (figure 5.8b). Or we can consider the ventral tissues from the diaphragm-to-psoas connection, along with the iliacus into the anterior adductors (pectineus, adductors brevis and longus), down behind the tibia and into the foot with the contents of the deep posterior compartment (figure 5.8c).

Diagnosis and Prescription—Pulsing

The fact that complex, long-chain movements require cooperation through many joints has been a theme through this text; we can now start to experiment with some movement principles in this exercise section.

To simultaneously engage all the tissues listed in the lunge position (a *range of movement*) requires enough *range of motion* at all the relevant joints, so that the strain can be distributed through each section relatively evenly. As we saw previously, this is true of any long-chain movement, and investigating the relationships between the ranges of motion is one of the main reasons to use these positions in the studio or clinic. The so-called "father of function," Gary Gray, would tell us that "every exercise is an assessment, and every assessment is an exercise."[4] I suggest that this true only if we *understand* what is happening through each joint range during a movement.

---

[4]Quote from one of his lectures.

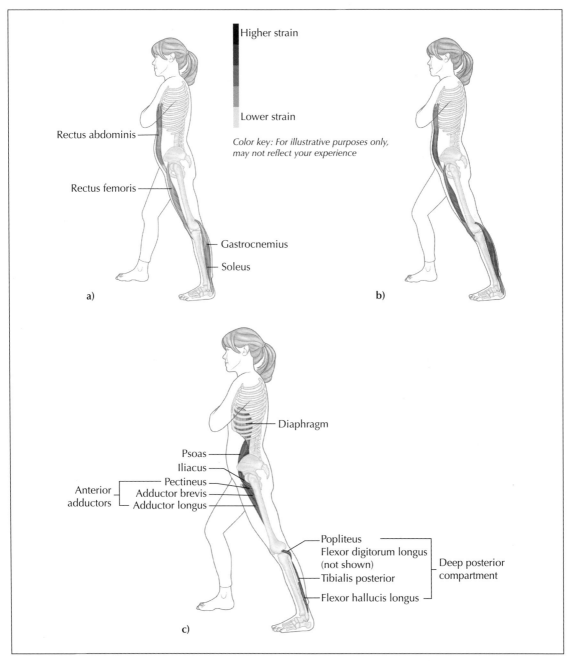

Higher strain

Lower strain

Color key: For illustrative purposes only, may not reflect your experience

Rectus abdominis

Rectus femoris

Gastrocnemius

Soleus

a)

b)

Diaphragm

Psoas

Iliacus

Pectineus

Adductor brevis

Adductor longus

Anterior adductors

Popliteus

Flexor digitorum longus (not shown)

Tibialis posterior

Flexor hallucis longus

Deep posterior compartment

c)

Figure 5.8. (a) The standard lunge position with the feet in parallel and the back leg straight lets us investigate the effects of a forward stretch into extension. (b and c) As the front knee moves forward, the client may feel a stretch in any number of tissues, as the joints of the back limb increase their range. The noncontinuous superficial tissues (b) include the rectus abdominis, rectus femoris, and the two main calf muscles, gastrocnemius and soleus. The ventral soft tissues are more likely to have more continuity, as their anatomy, actions, and positions all match to control the common joint couplings of ankle dorsiflexion and knee, hip, and spinal extension (c).

We can break down the movement joint by joint—or range by range, really, as it may not be the joint that limits the range of motion. Reduced or limited range across a joint can have numerous causes—soft-tissue tightness, previous injuries, or motor control inhibition, to name a few—and discovering the cause can be dependent on one's scope of practice. In general, provided there is no exacerbation of pain, no sense of bony restrictions (when it feels as though bone is hitting bone during movement), and no other obvious indication as to why putting strain into the area would cause damage, then using small-range, low-level pulsing movements can help mobilize the joint tissue and fluids, relax the muscle, and reassure a reluctant nervous system to "let it happen."

In their Fascial Fitness range of videos and courses, Robert Schleip and Divo Muller recommend gentle oscillations in and out of the end range. This highly effective approach not only helps increase range of motion but also improves tissue health and quality. Anyone can adopt that same principle using the positions shown in this text, as the positions are not only "stretches" or examples of movement possibility but are easily adaptable into powerful tools to improve health and vitality by incorporating gentle pulsing actions.

Slight bouncing actions in and out of end of range will:

- Stimulate fluid exchange—pushing water out and pulling it back in will increase tendon stiffness (which is a good thing!)
- Help align collagen fibers to increase their resiliency

- Stimulate mechanoreceptors and help regain trust in movement through the area.

These positive changes add up over time to create stronger, more elastic tissues around joints that have appropriate ranges of motion.

Pulsing the forward knee forward and back when in a lunge position can therefore become both diagnostic and therapeutic. The movement in and out of end range at each of the joints can expose where limitations might be held and, simultaneously, can help to unwind, release, or retrain any tissues that need gentle encouragement to "let go" into the movement. The gentle bouncing also provides some of the benefits listed above.

Assessment in each position is simply a matter of knowing which joint ranges should be involved with a movement and watching for their contributions. If a joint does not appear to be moving, we can change the exercise position or the direction of the movement, or change the environment for the client.

Coupling, Uncoupling, and Environmental Adjustments

The lunge-type position, and most other positions in this text, use simultaneous movement through several joints whose ranges are interrelated and often interdependent, or "coupled." To use the example of the lunge, ankle dorsiflexion, knee extension, and hip extension along the posterior lower limb must all have enough range to let the knee pulses have an effect through each joint. Reduced range in one of the joints will cause a reduction in the overall movement or a compensation strategy, or the movement will be focused only on the tissue associated with the limitation.

Learning to appreciate these relationships and see the patterns is a major aim of this text, so we will build the story steadily through each plane. Dividing the movements into the planes allows us the space and relative clarity for the practice and repetition that are necessary to become fluid with the "couplings" that act through the body.[5] Developing this new vision will be an incredibly powerful tool for analyzing movement and creating novel exercises and stretches, especially when dealing with compensation patterns.

For example, during long-chain movement we sometimes need to protect an area, perhaps because there was an injury, or maybe a surgical fixation has caused a limitation. Or maybe we want to bypass one area to focus more attention into another. In the example of the lunge position, limited ankle dorsiflexion can cause the back foot to turn out and the hip to receive a different line of stretch,[6] or it may reduce the overall range of movement.

If our aim is to create a line of strain through the tissue that *should* be involved with certain movements, then we might need a tissue-by-tissue strategy.[7] In this example, we can reduce the need for dorsiflexion range at the ankle by starting the movement from a more plantar flexed position. We could do that by placing a block of some form under the back heel, but often simply wearing a regular training shoe is enough (figure 5.9).

Footwear, bolsters, wedges, towels—almost anything you have to hand that provides a safe platform for the foot—can all be used for these slight adjustments. Making changes to the environment can add precision to movement, ensuring the strain gets to where it should go, and provides the client with even more information about how their body interrelates. Environmental adjustments can have the added benefit of helping you and the client monitor progress, as, gradually, if things are progressing in the right direction, the adjustments can be reduced or taken away altogether.

> *Evolution normally does not come to a halt, but constantly "tracks" the changing environment.*
>
> —**Richard Dawkins,**
> *The Blind Watchmaker*

Other environmental adjustments for different exercises can include positioning on angled surfaces, providing support for extra balance (such as a wall or holding onto a chair), or, when using the arms and hands during a movement, adding weight to the movement by holding dumbbells or bottles of water.

---

[5]I accept that "coupling" is a slight misnomer as there may be more than two joint ranges that are interrelated, but it is a word and concept that is familiar to most of us in the sense of interdependence.

[6]We will explore this later but try it for yourself now by performing the lunge stretch with your feet parallel, and then turn your back foot out 5°–10°. Can you feel how the stretch changes position in the back hip?

[7]The word "should" should be taken lightly, as there are probably many ideas of which tissues **should** be involved with any movement. And I **should** use fewer footnotes on any one page.

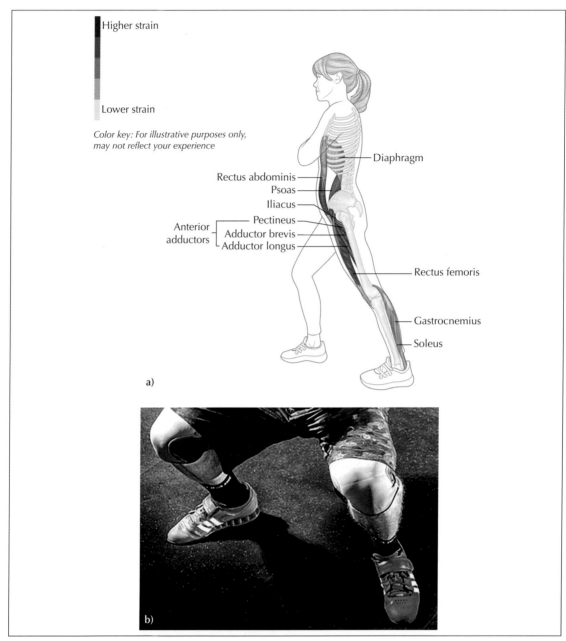

Higher strain

Lower strain

Color key: For illustrative purposes only, may not reflect your experience

Diaphragm

Rectus abdominis

Psoas

Iliacus

Pectineus

Anterior adductors — Adductor brevis

Adductor longus

Rectus femoris

Gastrocnemius

Soleus

a)

b)

Figure 5.9. (a) Most commercially available training shoes have some degree of height difference between the heel and the forefoot. Positioning the heel higher than the forefoot means that the ankle is relatively plantar flexed and starting the movement from plantar flexion can allow the tibia to tilt further forward, assisting the hip into extension. (b) This type of environmental adjustment is commonly used when lifting weights, where the knee must travel forward to keep the weight centered over the feet. Although the tibia will still be vertical, placing the feet in wedged shoes allows the tibia to start the movement forward from a relatively plantar flexed position.

However, adding weight will also increase the momentum of the movement and require monitoring the technique for any lack of control or areas of concern, especially when the movement includes spinal extension and rotations (figures 5.10–5.12).

For example, one assessment I often use early in a session is to have a client bring their arms up and almost straight back over their head (figure 5.10), because I want to see how the rib cage and spine react to the shoulder movement. The exercise is not precisely diagnostic, but it can reveal a lot about how a client organizes the relationship between their shoulders and their torso. Many people will hyperextend somewhere around the thoracolumbar junction (TLJ), which could indicate restricted thoracic extension or tightness/restriction around the shoulder tissues, especially the pectorals and the latissimus dorsi. In many cases I do not really need to know the cause, I just need to see the pattern and make adjustments to ensure safety during any other exercise that requires similar arm movements, especially if they are using weights.

A client's exaggerated spinal extension might be the result of a "movement groove," a habit, rather than any insult, injury, or dysfunction— it could be just how they organize their movement. The TLJ is an interface between the flexion/extension-dominant movement of the lumbars and the more three-dimensional, but extension-limited movement of the thoracics. It is important to keep in mind the many possible reasons why the thoracic spine and rib cage can be restricted. Not only are there many ligamentous and joint connections between

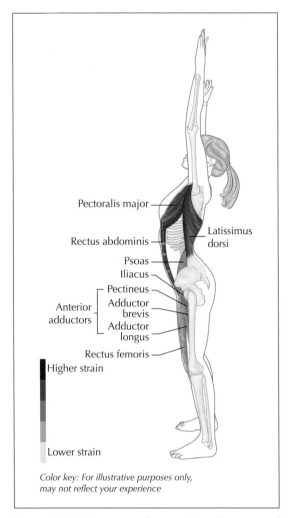

Color key: For illustrative purposes only, may not reflect your experience

Figure 5.10. It is common for people to hyperextend around the thoracolumbar area when taking their arms up and back. The movement does not reveal the source of the problem, but it should alert the therapist to watch for similar patterns and take care in other exercises that take the arms up and back, especially if using weights.

the ribs and vertebrae but the area can also be affected by changes to the breathing pattern, which can relate to emotional as well physical causes.

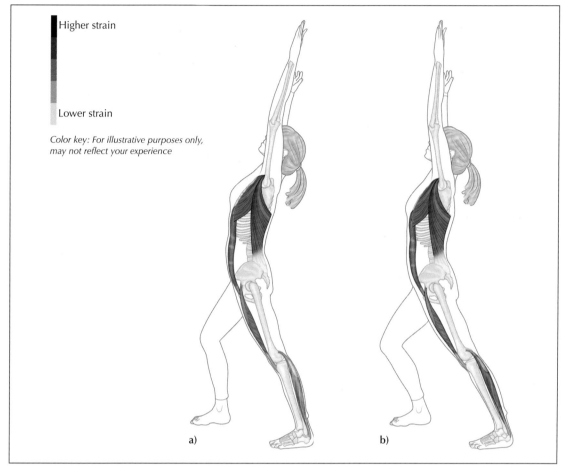

Higher strain

Lower strain

Color key: For illustrative purposes only, may not reflect your experience

a)

b)

Figure 5.11. (a) Pretensioning the anterior tissue by using the lunge position before they reach their arms overhead might help to support the client's back. (b) If the spine appears comfortable and supported, a knee driver, for example, could be used to increase the stretch along the front. The client could be asked to allow the head to tilt back (as shown), which is likely to increase the workload along the front of the body, or they may need to keep looking straight ahead to decrease the load and the extension in their spine.

Investigating all possible causes of restriction is beyond the scope of this short text, and, unless there are underlying pathologies, it is not necessarily essential for us to find out the specific cause in each individual's case. Provided due care and diligence are followed and the therapist stays within their scope of practice, the movements shown here should all be safe to perform. Our goals here are to normalize movement and improve overall capacity.

Increase Capacity and Look for Smoothness

Getting old is not a matter of age; it's a lack of movement. And the ultimate lack of movement is death.

—**Tony Robbins,**
Awaken the Giant Within

Our species has created an ecology for ourselves that our bodies are not adapted to—particularly when it comes to our lack of movement. Medicine has excelled in increasing the length of our lives, but government policies and our own personal choices have reduced its quality. Modern health-care systems are overburdened by cases of morbidity—the loss of health commonly brought about through the mismatch between the ecology our bodies evolved to thrive in and a modern lifestyle that tries to minimize our exposure to strain.

Despite knowing that our bodies are partly shaped through the work they do, we try to outsource that work to escalators, cars, and home-delivery pizza companies. With each of these choices we decrease our body's capacity for work and increase our chances of developing the diseases of morbidity, condemning ourselves to a long, uncomfortable, and slow demise. With better choices we can take advantage of our medical miracles by challenging our body to increase its capacity.

Increasing capacity for any client could relate to their breath and its tidal volume, their soft tissue's ability to deal with mechanical strain, or their muscle strength and power to lift more weight. These benefits and more will come through regular application of almost any movement practice.

However, movement practice should not be arbitrary. We need to address the "hinges" and "grooves," and the relatively overly mobile areas that might be taking more than their fair share of the strain during the exercises. By understanding the tools in this book—both the language that will help organize movement for you alongside the suggested movement repertoire—you will be ready to adjust the exercises to mobilize, train, stretch, open, support, or guide movement into the areas that crave it, or away from those that need protection.

My goal is not to teach a repertoire—there are enough of those already—the goal here is to understand anatomy in movement. If you have other skills, like the ability to cue clients clearly, or access to specialized equipment, use them. But do not fall back on the mindless following of some guru's ideas, or onto the aesthetics of what movement should look like. Let us get beyond "the rules" of movement and get excited by the living complexity that is the client in front of us.[8]

Helping the client reach their goals safely and effectively with support and perhaps some fun is the only *should* I should have to follow. Once I accept that as my guideline, then the world of movement is open to me. I can have my client place their feet where I want, move their hands

---

[8]You know "the rules"—all of those "shoulds" that we were taught. The knee *should* be …, the pelvis *should* be …, and the feet *should* maintain their tripod of support, and so on…

where I want, let their pelvis do what it wants—provided it is serving our primary goal. And, if my client has a tendency toward "hinging" when they take their arms up and back, then I can find a solution to help create smooth movement by thinking outside the box.

The containers, the stabilizers, and the guiding elements for that box are my client's system, and while that includes their emotions, psychology, and overall physiology, we must limit our descriptors here to their anatomy. Although that might sound restricting, it is much less so because we have removed those silly *rules of exercise.* By understanding anatomy and movement, my reference point for what is safe and appropriate now becomes my client. Their feet can go where they need to, their pelvis can do what it wants, their arms can swing around in any direction—if it helps serve our primary goal of increasing capacity and is safe.

For example, one of the indicators of a good back extension is the lack of hinging in any one area. Moving into extension requires the flexors to take much of the strain, especially if we use loading as the arms go back. Although these movements are often used to target the abdominals for eccentric loading, it is really *all* of the tissue in front of the spine that will be affected, and we would like *all* of it to do some work. We can enhance success and comfort in a movement by applying the information we explored in chapter 3—that pretension can help increase stability by putting the tissue in a position of advantage. We can apply that principle here to help support the spine during extension movements.

It might seem counterintuitive, but many clients can control spinal extension more easily when they are in the lunge position (figure 5.11). The foot position causes the pelvis to anteriorly tilt slightly, and the anteriorly tilted pelvis brings the lumbars into slight extension, thereby pretensioning the flexor tissues and preparing them for the eccentric work they are about to perform. Of course, not every client will feel this benefit. The lunge position might make some clients worse, while other clients may have to experiment to find the perfect distance between the front and back foot before we find their personal Goldilocks ratio, where the distance is neither too long nor too short, but is "just right."

The therapist and the client must feel free to experiment—no movement is presented to the client as *the* solution. The role of the therapist is to keep an open mind along with a watchful, knowing, observing, informed eye on our client as we ask them to move with different strategies.

Remember: "Every exercise is an assessment, and every assessment is an exercise."

Using Drivers to Change Direction

So far, we have used two movement drivers without labelling them as such—we used the knee to increase the stretch in the lunge position (figure 5.8) and we used the hands going overhead to discuss the role of the shoulder tissue in spinal extension (figure 5.10). A movement *driver* can be any body part, or even anything a client might be holding, that is cued to produce a movement reaction.

The list of what can be a driver is limited only by your imagination—hands, elbows, feet, and knees are the obvious and probably most common examples, but drivers could also include the nose, eyes, ears, shoulder, and sternum. Specific parts of the feet or hands, such as the heel, the thumb, or the "outside of the foot" could be used with the intention of creating a desired reaction or, importantly, assessing how the client reacts when using that driver.

> *Each one has to improve himself. Each driver has its limit. My limit is a little bit further than others'.*
>
> **—Ayrton Senna, interview after the 1988 Monaco Grand Prix**

Drivers can be used individually or in combination. There are no rules. The guidelines are to ensure safety and comfort for your client and then to pay attention and only increase difficulty and complexity once your client has achieved smoothness and competency with an easier exercise.

Sagittal Plane Movement and Rotational Motion

Most sagittal bilateral movements produce sagittal plane motions at the joints. We saw this with the flexion and extension reactions above. Because our limbs are off-center from the trunk, when one limb—upper or lower—is used as a driver it tends to introduce elements of rotation into the tissues.

Movements so far have used unilateral knee drivers for all the lunge movements and bilateral hand drivers for the overhead work. Now we can start to experiment and see what effects are created by using just one hand as the driver (figure 5.12). Experiment for yourself to find how your body reacts in the lunge position with the same-side arm and then the opposite-side arm driving back and overhead. Usually, when both limbs on one side are back (figure 5.12a), the response will be more sagittal. When the opposite limbs are back (figure 5.12b), more rotation is introduced into the movement.

Using Your Head

Some clients have a natural tendency to move their head with their movement and some do not—neither strategy is incorrect. Each option is just a different strategy that alters the tissue reaction. My most common approach is to simply ask a client to move whichever body part I have chosen as a driver and then watch what happens through their whole body. I observe their natural reaction, as this can give me information about how they would organize the movement in their normal life. If the client's first movement strategy is working for them, I let them carry on. If it looks hinge-like, creates discomfort, or if I need more information to clarify what is happening, then I will change the movement setup and instructions.

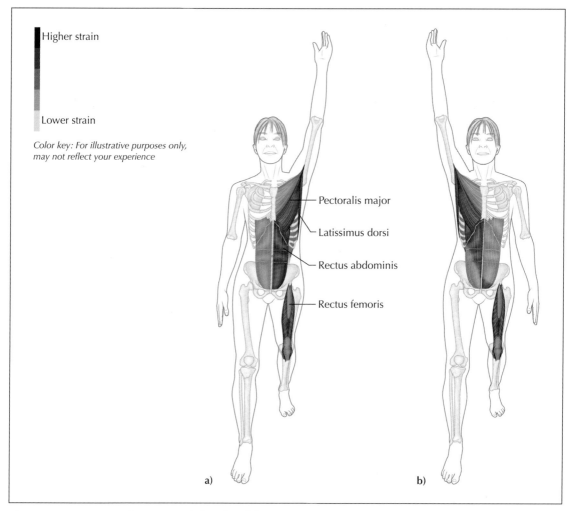

Higher strain

Lower strain

Color key: For illustrative purposes only, may not reflect your experience

Pectoralis major

Latissimus dorsi

Rectus abdominis

Rectus femoris

a)   b)

Figure 5.12. (a) Having the same-side hand and foot in a posterior position creates a vertical line of strain, in this case from the left shoulder to the left hip and thigh. (b) The opposite hand and foot in a posterior position causes a slightly oblique line of strain.

Changing Driver Angle—Using the Planes to Predict Reactions

> *Creativity arises from our ability to see things from many different angles.*
> —**Keri Smith, interview for *Wired***

The concept of movement drivers is an incredibly powerful tool for directing

movement to where it is needed, but the number of options can feel a little overwhelming at first. Returning to the basic principle of the relationship between the planes of movement and tissue reactions serves as a foundational framework to which we can keep coming back. Using the three planes gives us an organizational tool because, although the reaction created by each driver can vary through the body, we can use the sagittal, frontal, and transverse guidelines as rules of thumb to help organize our strategy.

As we saw earlier, movement in the sagittal plane leads to flexions and extensions, frontal plane movement causes side flexions, adductions, and abductions, while transverse plane movement relates to rotations. There are always slight variations and deviations that might happen because of joint type, injuries, or motor patterns, but keeping that rule of thumb in mind will help you orient to the first strategy when working with a client.

A simple cross-referencing system can then be put in place to match the driver, its direction, and the body's reaction. Working with flexor and extensor tissues will require sagittal plane movement—abductors and adductors react to frontal plane motion—and, obviously, the rotators relate to rotational motions. The straightforward correlation between joint actions, their corresponding soft tissues, and movement direction can form the basis of exercise prescription, and the correlation provides useful clues as to which muscles are active during normal movement—the flexors and extensors for sagittal plane movement, abductors and adductors for frontal plane motion, and the rotators for transverse plane motion.

Contrary to the impression given by some anatomy texts, the human body is not binary. Each muscle group does not work with a simple on-off—or agonist-antagonist—strategy. All muscles surrounding a joint work to stabilize, control, or create movement across the joint by adjusting their tension in relation to one another, placing more force where it is needed to create the desired or necessary outcome.

By adjusting a client's positioning, their movement drivers, and the direction of the driver, the therapist can create almost any movement reaction in the client's system to help retrain strength, control, or trust. Each movement option can be experienced and played with to let the therapist get a feel of what can happen in the client's system.

The choice of a driver for an exercise for a client will depend on the type of joint (hinge, ball-and-socket, condyloid, etc.), its alignment, and its health. When trying to choose exercise prescriptions, the many permutations can make it difficult to organize a client's movement suggestion quickly and usefully, but confidence builds quickly once the basic principles are in place.

Putting the Tools of the Trade into Action

We have covered many of the variables we can adjust—drivers (we have used the knee and the hands), foot position (which we have altered only once but will explore further in the next chapters), and the angle and direction of the drivers. Although this is not a long list, it already provides powerful tools for investigating and working with clients, as well as helping us understand the true tensegrity anatomy of the body.

As we have just mentioned, movement direction relates to the body's reaction, and, to take an example, we can explore what happens when a hand driver is used in different directions. When the hand is

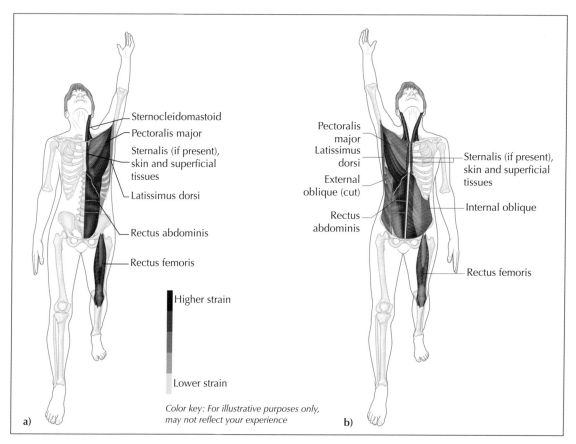

Figure 5.13. We can increase the load on the anterior tissues by allowing the head to move with the arm. Keep in mind that increasing the load requires increased attention from the trainer or therapist. Be sure you are observing from the sides and back as well the front view, as hinging in the back can be difficult to see from certain angles.

taken directly back over the shoulder, we see an almost purely sagittal plane reaction, as would be predicted (see figure 5.13a). However, that is not a common movement strategy; it is more likely that someone would take their arm back at a lower level, somewhere between the pure sagittal and transverse planes (figure 5.14).

A good tool improves the way you work.
A great tool improves the way you think.
—Jeff Duntemann,
Assembly Language Step-by-Step

Just like compass points, which blend the descriptions between north and west as north-northwest, northwest, west-northwest, we see a similar combination of "compass points" of the planes of motion happening as we change the angle of the arm. Straight over the shoulder leads to almost pure sagittal plane movement, taking the arm and hand straight back parallel to the floor (not shown, try it for yourself) will cause mostly rotation, and having your hand somewhere in between these two directions will give a combined extension/rotation (figures 5.14a and 5.15a).

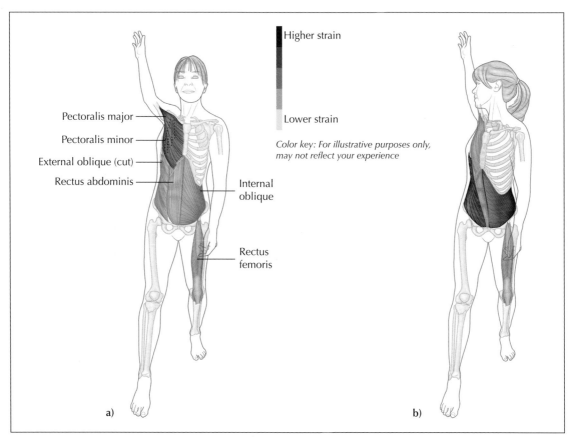

Higher strain

Lower strain

Color key: For illustrative purposes only, may not reflect your experience

Pectoralis major

Pectoralis minor

External oblique (cut)

Rectus abdominis

Internal oblique

Rectus femoris

a)

b)

Figure 5.14. A contralateral strategy (left leg back, right arm going back) is a safe and familiar position for most clients to start movement from, as it replicates many common movement patterns. Driving the arm back at an angle causes an extension-rotation reaction through the body and a stretch can be focused on the upper or lower trunk by looking straight ahead (a) or on the lower trunk by allowing the head to follow the arm (b).

Taking the experiment one step further, we can then use the head to change the tissue reactions. By letting the head follow the arm, the stretch is decreased in the upper body and focused more into the abdominals (figure 5.14b) or into the opposite adductors (figure 5.15b), depending on whether we use a contralateral or ipsilateral strategy (figures 5.14 and 5.15 respectively).

The choice to use contralateral, ipsilateral, head following, or head steady options in combination with the angle of the arm movement will relate to:

- The client's exercise goals
- Their performance demands (work or sport)
- Any "meaningful task" they have identified as part of the client interview (likely to relate to their performance demands)
- Their injury history:
  - We can explore the performance of affected tissue by putting some movement through the area.
  - We can protect it by reducing the movement demands.

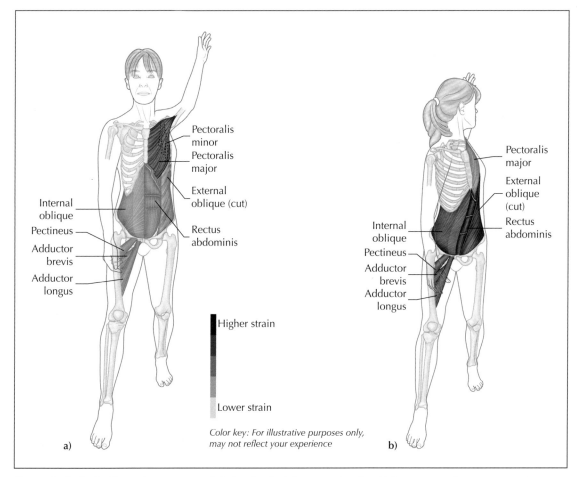

Figure 5.15. An ipsilateral movement (left leg back, left arm going back) is common in many sports, especially those involving a throwing action. A client's sport or work tasks might require them to either look at the target (head straight, a), or to look where their hand is reaching (head following, b), and so the movement strategy could be altered accordingly, and the reactive tissue strain will be different. When the head disassociates from the shoulder, the chest area is more likely to feel a stretch (a). When the head follows the arm, the thorax will also follow and come to a position where the shoulder, head, thorax, and pelvis are close to neutral to each other, and the strain is felt more in the adductors of the forward lower limb (b).

In addition:

- The client's age and overall strength and resilience will be a factor in how much loading we can use.

- Balance issues may affect their safety in using ipsilateral movement patterns.
- Probably many more factors will reveal themselves only when you have a client in front of you.

Going Forward—into New Explorations

Every movement modality has variations on forward bends. Whether it is "elephant" in Pilates or "downward dog" in yoga, these forward bends will all create strain along the back of the body. When done symmetrically, as most of them tend to be, they will create some degree of strain along that posterior line of tissue investigated by Vleeming in the early 1990s.

It can be interesting to play with adding asymmetry to a simple forward bend by using one hand as a driver for a forward and downward reach. Although we are presenting it as an exercise or stretch position, this action is a common everyday movement, such as when we bend forward to pick something up from a low shelf or from the floor. But this everyday movement has an important lesson to teach us regarding textbook muscle actions. Even though the hamstring stretch is probably one of the most common exercise and stretch actions, we rarely explore how the hamstring's angled approach from the leg to the ischium allows it to control hip rotation.

Most anatomy textbooks will tell us the hamstrings are hip extensors, knee flexors, and rotators of the knee when it is flexed. Rarely, if ever, do the textbooks mention that the hamstrings can also control hip rotation. To feel the hamstrings control hip rotation, try alternating between the positions shown in figures 5.16 and 5.17. With your left leg forward, take your right hand forward, down, and across to the left. Release slightly, then take your left hand forward, down, and across

to the right. Can you feel the change in tension between the medial (semitendinosus and semimembranosus) and the lateral (biceps femoris) hamstrings? If not, ask someone else to make the movement as you palpate their hamstrings, and watch what is happening at the hip as they reach forward, down, and across with alternating hands.

As the hand reaches from one side to the other, it causes the flexed hip to rotate slightly medially and then laterally. The degree of hip flexion is usually more or less the same, but it is the degree of rotation that is quite different, and you should be able to feel, either on yourself or with a partner, the effect rotation has on the line of strain.

How to Use the Movements

Despite the growing number of research papers showing the psychological, emotional, social, and physical benefits of movement, we still see many people choosing to avoid movement in all but essential forms. It is common in the complementary therapy world to bemoan this.

As manual and movement therapy teachers and practitioners, we need to find ways to empower clients back into a better relationship with their bodies and to find ways to bring movement back into their daily lives.

One reason for the body and mind to disconnect is because we outsource the responsibility for our own bodies. We want a doctor to be responsible for our health, we want a personal trainer to keep our fitness

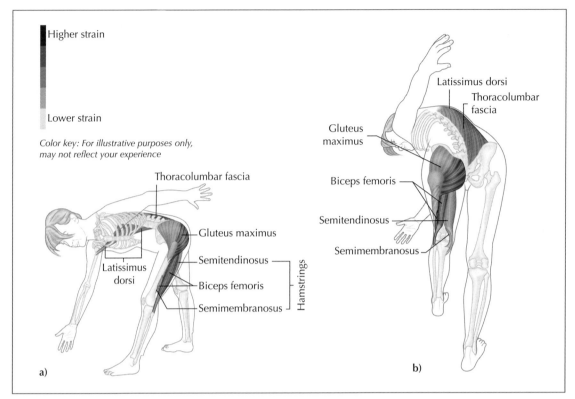

Figure 5.16. Using a contralateral strategy with one leg forward and the opposite hand reaching forward, down, and across causes the forward hip to flex, abduct slightly, and medially rotate. This movement will affect many tissues, including the myofascial continuity of gluteus maximus, thoracolumbar fascia, and opposite latissimus dorsi, as well as the hamstring control of hip rotation, creating more stretch into the biceps femoris.

on track, and we want the government to tell us what we should be doing—in essence, we line up the scapegoats to be blamed for our aches and pains. As part of this conspiracy, we allow the body to be looked at in sections, rather than as a whole, and most people do not realize that a problem in the hip is not a problem just of the hip but of a greater pattern.

The exercises in this chapter and those following can be used to help rebuild an understanding of the body's interrelated and interdependent truths. Even the simple lunge-type position can be used to demonstrate the relationship between the ankle and the hip, or the hip and the low back. Changing the movement drivers and their angles also highlights what happens in areas far from the part that is moving.

Every movement can be observed and adjusted to help reinforce the client's abilities and map their progress. Each movement position can be altered for the safety and comfort of the client, and the gentle pulses at the end of range can

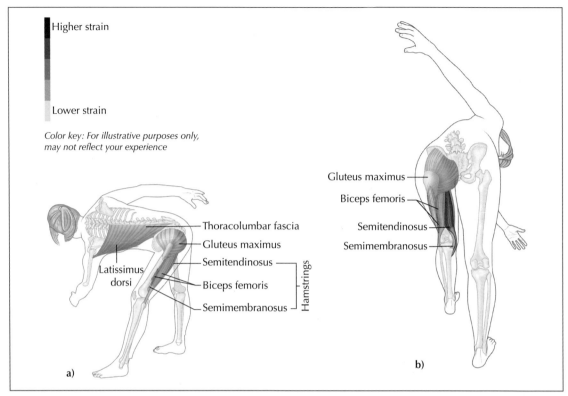

Higher strain

Lower strain

Color key: For illustrative purposes only, may not reflect your experience

Thoracolumbar fascia
Gluteus maximus
Semitendinosus
Biceps femoris
Semimembranosus
Hamstrings
Latissimus dorsi

Gluteus maximus
Biceps femoris
Semitendinosus
Semimembranosus

a)

b)

Figure 5.17. Using an ipsilateral strategy with one leg forward and the same-side hand reaching forward, down, and across causes the forward hip to flex, adduct slightly, and laterally rotate. This movement will have less effect on the myofascial continuity of gluteus maximus, thoracolumbar fascia, and opposite latissimus dorsi but might affect the posterior line a little more, and will create more stretch into the semimembranosus and semitendinosus.

be made low or high intensity by varying their speed, range, or load.

Of course, it is important to remain in your area of expertise, and dosage of the movements should be closely monitored. Two very useful guidelines are, firstly, to always start the session with a movement that is successful for the client, one that is easily replicated and performed to get them on the road to success and build their self-efficacy. The second is to monitor dosage of the movement by using only 5–10 pulses gently in and out of end range with an unloaded exercise. If you are trained to use loaded exercise, then you should have your own guideline, or follow Professor Stuart McGill's advice and stop your client on the first repetition that shows a negative change of form.

The overall aim is to increase the client's self-efficacy—their confidence that they can move, that they have a body that works, and that they can use it to recapture some of the joy and fun of life. We want to decrease morbidity and help clients regain a sense of themselves.

Summary

These exercises and movements can be performed for self-exploration or as therapeutic tools. They are not just about increasing ranges of movement and motion but explorations in connectivity of the body that are useful for learning functional anatomy and for learning how bodies interrelate during movement.

By taking control of positioning and movement drivers we can create relatively predictable reactions through the body. This chapter has investigated sagittal plane relationships and the effects of offset foot positions, and the differences between same-side and opposite-side limb movements. One-sided drivers introduced some rotation to movement, especially when using the upper limb, which has a wider movement range than the lower limb, which is commonly rooted to the floor, limiting its axis of movement to the predominately sagittal talar joint of the ankle and the knee joint.

We have also learned to change the focus of strain through the body by having the head remain still or track the arm movement. Having the head and arm move together moved much of the strain below the thorax compared with when the head was looking forward, which then encouraged the thorax to stay in place.

Through the simple manipulation of drivers and directions we can be quite accurate in how strain is experienced through the body. Adjusting movement through these tools can help target areas that may benefit from more or—importantly—less strain, as we try to ensure the smooth and consistent contributions from each joint and tissue through the movement strain.

Although the chapter focused mostly on sagittal plane motions, we took the "liberal" interpretation of the plane and made numerous off-center adjustments. Using the lunge-type position allowed us to access contralateral movement patterns and exposed hamstring actions that are rarely discussed.

The rotational control of the hip by the hamstrings is not something I have ever read in a textbook, but it is clearly felt during the movement. This kind of "reverse action" is commonly overlooked owing to our tendency toward concentric actions—these and many more revelations will come to you as you work through the exercises.

Reflection Questions

1. What is the difference between the anterior/posterior body and the ventral/dorsal aspects?
2. What do you understand about the relationship between soft-tissue alignment and joints?
3. How are ankle, knee, and hip joint movements "coupled" during skipping, jumping, and running?
4. How many drivers can you think of that could be used to create flexion of your right hip?
5. Why is sagittal plane movement so closely related to rotations?

Notes

In his recent book *Exercised: Why Something We Never Evolved to Do Is Healthy and Rewarding* (Knopf Doubleday, 2021), Professor Daniel Lieberman explains the growing gap between what our bodies have evolved to do and what we actually experience day to day. Survival is a matter of balancing the simple equation of using fewer calories than we can put into our system. Lieberman points out it is therefore natural and even adaptive for us to want to save calories and that exercise is an unusual thing to want to do.

Few people in the West have to search and struggle to gather food, so few calories are used in the hunting and gathering process; we also design our days to minimize movement by using cars, elevators, and all manner of labor-saving devices. Not only are we growing obese but we are also under-stimulating our bodies, which require stress to develop muscle.

The resultant muscle weakness (especially the sarcopenia caused by aging), loss of range of motion, and reduced cardiorespiratory fitness all go to increase the general lack of health toward the end of life—and though life may be extended through medical intervention, it is likely to lack quality and depth.

Therapies often focus on the reduction of pain—I think that is missing the point. We should also focus on improved quality of life. One way is to encourage clients to re-friend their body through movement to retain muscle strength, along with quality and range of motion.

Moving to the Side

*It's just a jump to the left
And then a step to the right
Put your hands on your hips
You bring your knees tight*
—**Richard O'Brien, "Time Warp"**

Introduction

We tend to be more familiar with flexion-extension relationships in the body than with how side flexion, adduction, or abduction travels through the body. It seems obvious that when we bend a knee forward, the other joints above and below will also move in a similar way. We are comfortable with the idea of our bodies as continuous structures with joints that let us flex and extend. But when we come to the other planes, that expectation somehow gets lost, or at best the understanding of what should happen becomes fuzzy. We will start to put that right by exploring frontal plane relationships in this chapter and continue to the transverse plane in the next.

I am sure part of the reason for the fuzziness around frontal plane movement is the way

we apply our understanding of anatomy to the creation of exercises. What would our exercises look like if we started from an appreciation of normal, everyday movement instead of from textbook anatomy? This chapter will explore the full body's "tensegrity-based" reaction to side-to-side movement. We will see that it follows a very similar pattern to the sagittal plane reactions we saw in chapter 5, but this time the language changes from flexions and extensions to side flexion in the spine, adduction and abduction through the limbs, and inversion and eversion of the subtalar joints.

Although mentioned before, it is still worth repeating that each plane of movement has a corresponding terminology for the reactions at the joints. Sagittal plane movement is all about flexion and extension, while frontal plane movement is all about side flexion, the forever-muddled abduction and adduction, and inversion and eversion. In contrast to the many words for frontal plane motion, the transverse plane requires only one—rotation. We will continue to explore this relationship between movement direction and joint reaction below, and see how we can use our

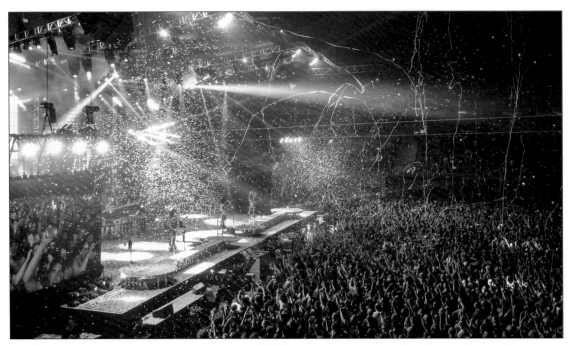

Figure 6.1. Let yourself reminisce about the good old days when rock stars were rock stars, the music was interesting, and though the band played hard, everyone got to show their soft side during the power ballad. As you wave the imaginary lighter in the air, let your body sway back and forth with it, and then pause at either side to feel what has happened through the major joints. At the end of your comfortable "side-to-side" range, can you list most of the joint reactions?

vision of a movement to predict and describe the joint reactions.

First, let's explore what happens with the large, full-body frontal plane movements and how they track through body.

Frontal Plane Movement

> *Progression is going forward. Going backward is regression. Going sideways is just aggression.*
> —**Noel Gallagher,** *Belfast Telegraph*

Just as we did with the sagittal plane, let's begin our frontal plane journey with an overhead movement—some readers might remember this move from the obligatory power ballad moment during any 1980s rock concert, when we would all light a lighter (when such things were commonplace and allowed in concert halls!) and sway it side to side above our heads in time to the music (figure 6.1).

As mentioned above, the frontal plane movement vocabulary includes side flexion, abduction and adduction, and inversion and eversion, and this simple but full-body movement has them all. As descriptors, side flexion is used only for spinal motion, inversion and eversion take place at the subtalar joint, but abduction and adduction occur through many joints and joints of different types.[1]

Full-body frontal plane movement will cause the spine to side flex and the hips to abduct on one side and adduct on the other, while one subtalar joint inverts and the other everts. Spinal side flexion is quite straightforward and provides few surprises, but the relationships at the hips and ankles are worth spending some time over, as we tend to be less familiar with these left and right, or opposite-side, relationships.

We make many movements that require the pelvis to tilt during our normal daily activities (figure 6.2a). Walking is the obvious and most common example, but others, such as reaching for the top shelf, cleaning the top window, or preparing to get up from the seat of a bus will all request different actions from each hip joint. Of course, we may not be in the "frontal plane neutral" of anatomical position when that happens, and so the hip may be in some combination of flexion and rotation. The complexity of those movements brings us back to a reminder of how we are using the vocabulary in combinations to facilitate comparisons and to place anatomy in context—the words exist to empower us and assist our perception and should not be limited to the restricted fantasy world of single-axis movement.

We tend to invent exercises that work the abductors and adductors in open-chain movement with the lower limbs free to move toward or away from the midline independently or in unison. However, once our feet are on the floor and the "chain" is closed, it is the pelvis that moves over the legs, and, as it travels to the side, one hip adducts as the other one abducts.

Changing from open- to closed-chain motion means the muscle actions change from a concentric action that creates the motion during open-chain movement to an eccentric control when performing closed-chain movements. To put this in context, look at the clamshell exercise in figure 1.6a, in which the abductors of the hip joint are shortening—the concentric action of the gluteus maximus. Then contrast that with the right hip of the woman walking in figure 1.6b. The right hip is adducting, and that motion requires control and deceleration—the eccentric action of gluteus maximus (among other muscles).

It is true that the clamshell also requires muscles to work eccentrically when the knee is controlled downward to meet its counterpart on the floor, but the muscles are still controlling movement of the femur. When the pelvis tilts during closed-chain motions, the abductors need to control the pelvis more than the femur. While this might seem like nit-picking, it is important to break the common—often unconscious—prejudices with which we interpret anatomy.

As mentioned earlier, anatomy teaching provides us with lots of information but not all of it is useful for interpreting normal movement. Many references still use "origins"

---

[1] While the ball-and-socket joints of the glenohumeral and hip joints might be best known for ab/adduction, the fingers and toes can also abduct and adduct at the metacarpo- and metatarsophalangeal joints owing to the condyloid joint arrangement. This movement pattern also results from the vertebrate body plan, which tends to draw inward in flexion (flex and adduct) and expand out in extension (extend and abduct).

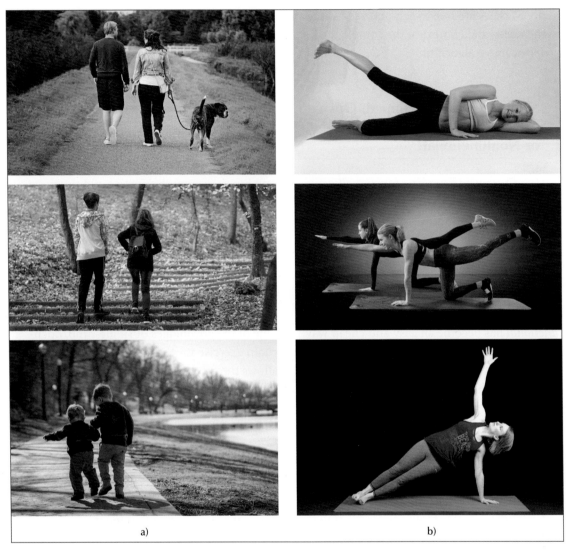

Figure 6.2. Normal, everyday movement tends to be asymmetrical at the hips. (a) Walking, among many other activities, causes the pelvis to tilt side to side, with the hips adducting and abducting on opposite sides. (b) Everyday, closed-chain movements with the feet on the floor contrast with many mat and equipment exercises that are either unilateral or symmetrical.

and "insertions" and, even if they have dropped the silly idea that insertions *always* move toward origins, the lists of actions given in every textbook and asked of us for exams are based on the same incorrect and limiting assumptions, relating to anatomical neutral and concentric actions. The ability

to *see* anatomy benefits from accepting that muscles can act at either end—and they will act to *provide*, *control*, or *prevent* movement, depending on the needs of the task.

Thankfully, muscles have not read the anatomy books and do not know what they are *supposed* to do. Muscles are free to respond according to the needs and context of the complicated proprioceptive algorithm.

Single- or Double-Hipped, Open or Closed Chain, Functional or Nonfunctional?

Customers want new functionality, but they don't want the traditional complexity that has marred products in the past.
—**Marc Benioff,** *Behind the Cloud*

Attacking or undermining certain exercises because they are deemed more or less *functional* has become an easy and cheap way to attract attention on social media platforms. Some trainers have used this scapegoating, headline-grabbing, and provocative strategy as a deliberate way to build a following, but it only alienates others and demonstrates their own lack of understanding. As we mentioned before, what makes an exercise functional or not functional is not anything inherent within the exercise itself but is in the trainer's understanding of how that exercise fits into the scheme for building success for the client.

Keep in mind that the movements shown through this text are not here because they are the best, most challenging, most fascial, most functional, or most ..., whatever the trend will be whenever you are reading this book. The exercises and movements are here because they help you build an understanding of how the body relates through itself so that you can better interpret a client's movement pattern and break out of generic prescription-based protocols that don't work for everyone. While single-joint exercise is not our focus here,

please keep in mind that it certainly has its place in helping people build up to complex movements, to develop focused strength and range of motion, and to improve the quality of connection and control in that area.

Due to its range of motion, the hip is a great place to investigate some of the complexities of movement and we will explore direction and hip movement below to build the three-dimensional model in our minds. As a ball-and-socket joint, the hip joint has one of the widest ranges available in the body, but the range available at one hip can depend on what is happening in the rest of the body, especially around the other hip.

One of the advantages of single-limb, open-chain exercise for the lower limb is that it allows the hip to move as much as it can, as the couplings between the femur and pelvis to other joints are lessened, if not removed altogether. For example, stand on one leg and swing the other in as wide an arc as possible and then try standing on both legs and move the pelvis over the leg—it is impossible to move the hip through the same range of motion when moving the pelvis in closed-chain. Later we will see the significant relationships and couplings between the hips, the trunk, and even the arms when we look at the hip joint in its wider context.

Long-Chain Movement—the Importance of Essential Events and Coupling

In chapter 4 we introduced the concept of "coupling" to explain how in some areas, in some movements, the range of motion at two or more joints is interdependently linked, and we explored the effects of coupling with the relationship between ankle dorsiflexion and knee and hip extension during a lunge. A restriction at one of these sites influences the others because in normal life—as well as sports—the completion of a task is of utmost importance. The body has ways of working around limitations, and successful execution of a throw, catch, kick, or run is something we will make sacrifices for—and too often that sacrifice is of tissue integrity.

I find it useful to break down complex movements into manageable chunks. What should happen at each joint if, for example, I want to reach and lift my coffee with my right hand.[2] If we know which body part is moving, what direction it is moving in, and roughly how far it is moving we should be able to work out which joints should be reacting and in what direction they should be moving. And, if we know which joints should be moving, we can take a good stab at guessing which soft tissues are involved in the creation, control, or inhibition of the movement.

Try it for yourself—how many strategies to reach your hand forward can you discover?

Can you add any to the list below?

> If you are seated, you could bend at the hips.
> You could use almost pure shoulder protraction.
> You could isolate your glenohumeral joint.
> You could flex and rotate your thoracic spine.

The answers might depend on where exactly the cup is positioned and how much range you have available in each of these areas. A limitation in one area can necessitate an increase in another, and any combination of the above strategies would also get the job done. Most of us should be able to experiment with each of these strategies, but what if you have only one or two of them available to you every day? What if—rather than the easy task of lifting a coffee cup—the movement was much larger with greater forces involved? Would you want to always use the same few tissues?

Most people would agree that force should be spread through as many tissues as appropriate to achieve the task at hand. We don't want to repeatedly overload a few tissues or limit the work to the same muscles and tissues each time. I use the term "essential events" to communicate the idea of appropriate tissue contribution during any movement. Any movement can be broken down into a series of "events" through the body, each of which should contribute appropriately toward the successful execution of the movement.

But what does "appropriate" mean? How many tissues are appropriate? And, to what degree should they be strained? These are important questions that can be answered only in the context of a client, their medical history, their desired movement goal, and their tissue type, among many other variables. We will start by developing the language and the vision to break down what should happen during any long-chain movement.

To help embed the difference between coupling and essential events, return to the example of reaching for the cup of coffee. Depending on the distance between your

---

[2] Nowadays, that task is still within my achievable range. It's a long time since I performed a competitive throw, catch, kick, or run.

hand and the cup, the task could be performed using any one of the listed strategies because, within a short range of motion, none of the motions is coupled to any other in the list. All of the cup-reaching strategies can be broken down into a series of essential events, but none of the joint movements (essential events) involved is coupled to another. The coffee cup reach contrasts with the lunge position we explored in chapter 5, in which ankle,

knee, and hip are all interdependent and are therefore "coupled."

Now we have some more movement vocabulary under our belts, let's come back to the first example in figure 6.1b, as this will help us see the relationship between the two hip joints and the low back (figure 6.3). This triangle of joints and tissues is interdependent (i.e., coupled), and any restriction or limitation

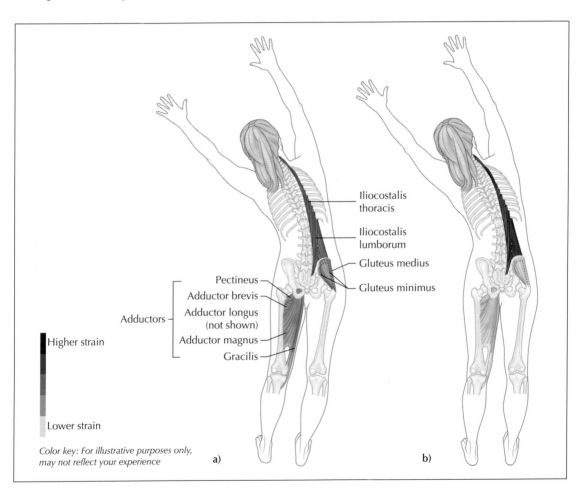

Figure 6.3. (a) As we swing our arms to the left, the right hip abductors, left hip adductors, and the lower right spinal muscles have to work eccentrically to control the movement as it happens. (b) If one of those areas is weak or restricted for any reason (here, the right abductors), the motion at each of the others will be reduced unless a compensation strategy is found. In this example, left hip abduction has been limited by the lack of movement in the right hip but the reduced ranges of motion in the hips have been compensated for by increasing spinal side flexion.

at one will have a knock-on effect on the others. Try it: stand up and swing your arms as you did before, allowing your body to respond naturally. Then try to do the same movement without letting your right hip adduct as your arms swing left, then without letting your left hip abduct, and a third time, not letting your low back side bend. It doesn't matter which of the three movement ranges is taken away, the others also reduce.

The joint and soft-tissue triangle responsible for hip abduction, opposite side hip adduction, and lower lumbar side flexion is coupled. The removal of one range of motion directly affects the others. In this case, the ranges are all reduced because of the nature of the functional connections between. But that is not always the case.

During other long-chain movement there will be many joint ranges that are not coupled together, allowing one joint to increase its range to compensate for a reduction elsewhere.

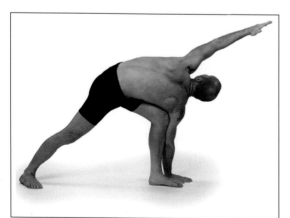

Figure 6.4. In real life, it is our overall range of movement that matters, and we pay little attention to the range of motion at individual joints. It can be very informative for therapists to watch for areas of relative hyper- and hypomobility when clients are making a long-chain movement.

For example, the reduced motion in the hip and low back (figure 6.3b) could be compensated for by increasing the ranges of motion above or below the restricted area. This is especially true in real-life movement, when people can often be seen compensating for restrictions in one part by overreaching in others, an action that you might recognize in many stretching and yoga-type classes (figure 6.4).

Range of Motion and Range of Movement

My definition of elegance is the achievement of a given functionality with a minimum of mechanism and a maximum of clarity.
—**Fernando J. Corbató, "On Building Systems that Will Fail"**

How do we define "elegance"? We recognize beautiful movement when we see it, but what qualities are present that make it stand out? One aspect is the distribution of strain through the body—we don't want to see angles and hinges in the body—we watch contortionists for that visceral squeeze they evoke. Differentiating between ranges of motion and range of movement is useful for analyzing everyday movement and helps us verbalize the qualities of minimum mechanism and maximum clarity.

Most everyday tasks are long-chain movements that involve contributions from numerous joints. These tasks require us to get some part of our anatomy to somewhere, usually while another part is anchored somewhere else. Our feet can be planted on the floor, our pelvis on a seat, or our back against a chair as we reach our hand out for that ever-tempting coffee cup. Each joint between the fixed point and the moving limb (or desired end goal) could be involved in the movement, and each joint can provide something toward the overall range of movement. The *range of movement* is therefore the range from the fixed point to the destination of your hand—the coffee cup.

Each joint between the two points—the "fixed" and the "destination"—can contribute a portion of its *range of motion*. The overall movement is an accumulation of those contributions, which can vary for many reasons. These may be the nature of the movement, the design of the joint, the environment, motor control differences, injury history—even the perceived aesthetics of movement will affect which tissues move more or move less. Every possible reason for any limitation or reduction should be investigated through appropriate history taking, isolated joint testing (if within your skill set), or focusing gentle movement through that area to see what happens.

And now, time to start putting it all together.

Any long-chain movement has beginning and end points that require the ability to achieve the *range of movement* between them. A smooth and distributed execution of that movement will require numerous *essential events* in the tissues between the two points. Each joint should contribute an appropriate *range of motion* to allow the soft tissues to work within their optimal, efficient range for that task. Some joints might not be able to contribute because of injury or motor control changes, or because they are *coupled* to other,

limited, joints that prevent them from reaching their working range of motion.

The above paragraph might seem a little jargon-heavy at first, but reread it and then work through the rest of the text. Keep the concepts in mind as you try out the exercises, and you will see their purpose and their power. Getting to grips with these concepts will improve your vision and understanding.

> This is a good opportunity to go back to chapter 5 and review some of the concepts there. Have a look at figure 5.10—what are the *essential events* through that movement?
>
> The *range of movement* appears to be normal, but the body position lacks smoothness. Where are the imbalances between individual joint and tissue *ranges of motion*?
>
> Now work through some of the other exercises from chapter 5 and experiment with the language. Pay particular attention to which joints are contributing to the overall movement. Are any of them linked in ways that might indicate they are *coupled*?

Side Flexion and Myofascial Continuity

First impressions are always unreliable.
—**Franz Kafka**

In the last 20 years, the idea of myofascial continuity has been popularized but not properly considered from a functional point of view. The idea of a "lateral line" from feet to head has entered into many movement repertoires, with the claim of continuity between the hip abductors and the abdominal obliques on the same side of the body. However, a continuity that allows transfer of force between these two areas does not make sense for our normal movement patterns. Long-chain side flexion, such as in figure 6.3, is quite uncommon outside of gyms and yoga and Pilates studios. We are more likely to lengthen the abductors on one side as we lengthen the abdominals on the other side—the kind of daily movements seen in figure 6.2a.

As the pelvis tilts side to side (e.g., in walking), one hip adducts, the opposite side abducts, and this movement requires control of the pelvis from above the iliac crest on one side and below it on the other side (figure 6.5a). The iliac crest will be moving away from the greater trochanter on the side that is adducting, and, as we discussed above, the muscle tissue between those points will control this closed-chain movement. This myofascial tissue will require a strong degree of anchorage on the inferior iliac crest to perform its task.

On the other side, the ilium is moving down and away from the rib cage, so it benefits from the strong attachment of the abdominal muscles on top of the iliac crest. It is rare that we side flex in the frontal plane—that movement is mostly limited to exercise classes and anatomy books. It is much more common to have some degree of rotation between the ribs and the ilium as the ilium drops away—and now the obliques finally make sense (figure 6.5b). The obliques are not just for rotational crunches. Their functional role is to help control the movement of the pelvis away from the ribs (and vice versa!) when there is rotation between the two parts. It does not matter whether the

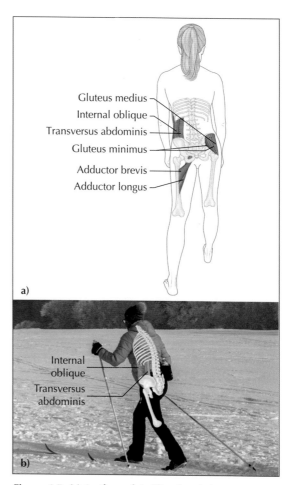

a)

b)

Figure 6.5. (a) As the pelvis tilts, the abductors on one side control adduction through their connection to the inferior aspect of the iliac crest. On the other side of the pelvis, the abdominal obliques attach to the superior aspect of the iliac crest and therefore help decelerate the drop of the ilium. It would not make sense to allow the obliques and abductors to transfer force between each other on the same side as it would inhibit their ability to manage pelvic tilts. (b) Most functional movements create some degree of rotation between the rib cage and pelvis. Having the lateral abdominals angled allows them to control both the side tilt and the rotational aspect of the movement, whether the pelvis is behind the rib cage (as shown) and controlled by the internal obliques or in front and controlled by the external obliques (not shown, but you get the idea).

pelvis is in front or behind, there will be a fiber direction to help control the movement.

Many people claim to feel the "myofascial connection" along the lateral line during side bends. This is a problem not of sensation but of vocabulary and sense of depth. As we saw in the discussion of the superficial front line, continuity of the myofascia is not essential to transfer force between two structures, and we should keep in mind that continuity does not prove transfer of force, nor does transfer of force prove myofascial continuity.

Force transfer might benefit from direct continuity between structures, but it is not dependent upon it. Once again, we need to appreciate the importance of understanding movement first and then seeking to relate the patterns to anatomy, rather than the other way round. The outcome of "anatomy stories" is that many people started to perform "lateral line myofascial stretches" when no such thing really exists nor serves much real-life functional purpose.

Side flexing from anatomical position will create strain along the lateral aspect of the body, primarily in the skin and the layers most closely associated with it (figure 6.6). This is especially true when the side flexion is performed with the arm abducted, an action that creates even more superficial strain along the lateral aspect.[3] In conversation with bodyworkers and movement therapists, Adjunct Professor Laurice Nemetz and Gary Carter (leading dissectors of the Fascial Net Plastination Project) both agreed that the

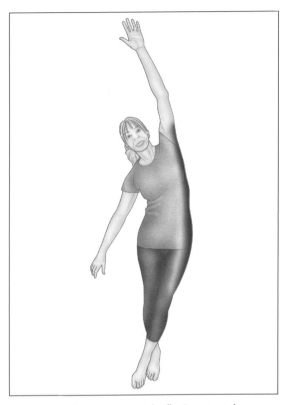

Figure 6.6. The common side-flexion stretch has been associated with proposed myofascial continuity along the lateral aspect, but the strain is much more likely to be carried by superficial fascial layers, including the skin, rather than by the deeper muscles.

deeper layers of the myofascia are strongly connected to the bone either side of the iliac crest. The gluteal muscles attach below and the abdominals attach above the line of bone, with little to no direct fascial connection between them. In contrast, the superficial layers of skin and adipose tissue have much more freedom to glide back and forth across the crest.

Increased strain along the lateral skin and adipose tissue is likely to create the sensation of stretch, and few people argue about the skin's continuity over the iliac crest. The superficial tissues can move and glide over

---

[3] Please remember, *strain* refers only to the change in tissue length, and should not be read as the perception of increased tension that we often associate with it.

the iliac crest—something that the deeper, underlying myofascia of the obliques and hip abductors cannot do.

Peeling the Onion Skin— Layered Anatomy

Understanding the implications of layered anatomy can be incredibly useful if we want to target certain myofascial tissues. For example, many references show the side-flexion stretch as a method to target the quadratus lumborum, but there are a few problems with this. When performing the stretch, many people will give an extra reach of their hand to "feel the stretch" and "really open up." But the extra reach of the hand is more likely to cause more strain in the superficial tissues and would probably inhibit the strain coming into the deeper quadratus lumborum.

You can feel this easily for yourself with the simple exercise shown in figure 6.7. The upward reach of the arm

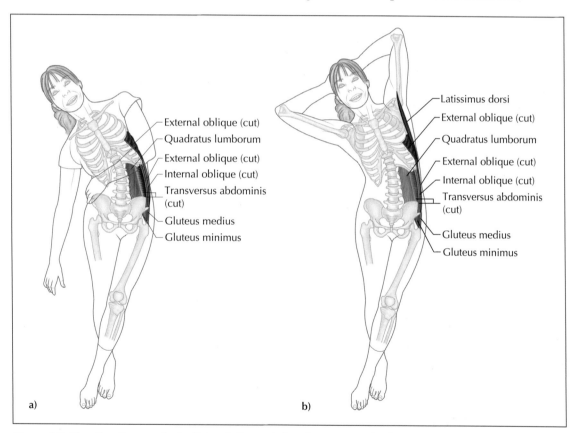

a)

External oblique (cut)
Quadratus lumborum
External oblique (cut)
Internal oblique (cut)
Transversus abdominis (cut)
Gluteus medius
Gluteus minimus

b)

Latissimus dorsi
External oblique (cut)
Quadratus lumborum
External oblique (cut)
Internal oblique (cut)
Transversus abdominis (cut)
Gluteus medius
Gluteus minimus

Figure 6.7. Elevating the arm (as in figure 6.6) may bring the strain to the level of the skin, but it can also help support the body by adding pretension along the lateral aspect. (a) Using a downward reach of the opposite side arm may reduce the skin stretch and bring the strain to deeper levels, but it might create instability and focus the stretch between the ribs and the pelvis rather than into the lateral abductors. (b) Having the hands behind the head may be a useful compromise between providing enough stability to let the pelvis tilt and not overstretching the superficial tissues.

tensions the superficial tissues first, including the latissimus dorsi and the lateral abdominals. When most people repeat the exercise without the arm elevated, it gives a larger range of side flexion but with a reduced sense of "stretch"—probably indicating that the strain in the first movement isn't able to reach or affect the quadratus lumborum.

However, performing the side flexion without the arm abducted can feel quite unstable for many people. The instability can be due to the increased range of movement, which brings the center of gravity further away from the center of support and forces the deeper muscles to work harder without the extra support of the superficial tension. This leaves us in a quandary—how do we "stretch" the quadratus lumborum without creating instability? We could experiment by having the hands behind the head (figure 6.7b). This half-abducted shoulder position might create enough strain in the superficial tissues to support the movement without reducing the range so much that the movement doesn't reach the deeper layers.

Direction—Bottom-Up or Top-Down?

We worry top-down, but we invest bottom-up.
—**Seth Klarman,** *Margin of Safety*

Most side-flexor stretches are performed in the anatomy-book-friendly direction—top-down—and have created much confusion about side flexion and quadratus-lumborum-focused movements. These problems are driven by our bias toward anatomical position and open-chain-movement ideas. It is true that quadratus lumborum and its associated side flexors will create and control spinal side flexion as performed in the exercise in figure 6.7, but in everyday life they will also regularly be involved in side flexion of the spine driven upward from the pelvis.

Reversing movement direction can sometimes pay huge dividends by facilitating more accuracy and being more functional, and it creates more variety and interest. Some of that heightened interest is the new depth it can give to our understanding of soft tissues. For example, we looked at pelvic tilt in response to functional movement above, seeing how the "functional triangle" between the abductors and adductors of the opposite hips work in conjunction with the lower fibers of the quadratus lumborum (along with some of the abdominals; see figures 6.2a and 6.5). Anatomy books rarely show or discuss the different alternating fiber directions of quadratus lumborum (QL), leaving most of us with the image of a predominantly vertical orientation, but now we can appreciate the functionality of those lower fibers (figure 6.8).

The presence of the iliolumbar (up and in from the ilia to the transverse processes) and the lumbocostal (up and out from the transverse processes to the lower ribs) fibers of the QL is contested by some anatomists, but in practice their objections are meaningless. The truth is that we have to control spinal side flexion from different directions whether we have these obliquely oriented QL fibers or not. Whether a client has those exact fibers present or missing is a question we will probably never know the answer to—and the answer makes

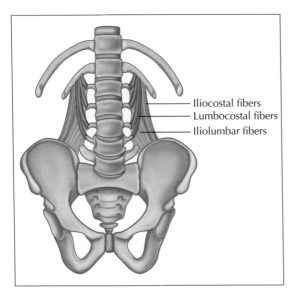

Iliocostal fibers
Lumbocostal fibers
Iliolumbar fibers

Figure 6.8. Most of us are familiar with the representation of the quadratus lumborum (QL) shown in green, and the vertical alignment matches with our image of its involvement with spinal side flexion. However, some research papers show that the QL also has fibers that travel up and in from the ilium to the lumbar vertebrae (in yellow), and up and out from the lumbar vertebrae to the twelfth rib (in purple).

no difference to how we should approach their functional ability. We know that most people will side flex their lower ribs away from the lumbars when they reach across to grab their coffee, and we know that their pelvis will tilt downward away from the lumbars as they walk away from the counter. It is these functional ranges that we should work on—not the "anatomy stories" that we impose on ourselves.

Awareness of the direction the reactions are traveling through the body is a very useful skill. Changing between top-down and bottom-up movements allows you to adjust and fine-tune the focus of many exercises and stretches, and it can be vital in understanding

how the body is reacting during complex movements. In the case above, we can use the anatomy story of the different angles of the QL to remind us to change the order and direction in which we enter various stretches. Moving the rib cage first, either by the reach of the hand or the simple tilt of the ribs or head, is more likely to influence the upper lumbocostal area—a top-down reaction. Whereas starting a movement from the lower limb or pelvis may target the iliolumbar fibers more effectively—a bottom-up reaction.

Increasing Capacity

Life isn't about finding yourself. Life is about creating yourself.
—George Bernard Shaw,
An Unsocial Socialist

There are many myths and a lot of accumulated confusion and quite a few frustrations when it comes to understanding exactly what is happening with soft tissues when we "stretch" and "work" them. We will leave those anatomy stories to one side and confine our exploration to what happens when we move in certain directions and whether we can focus an intention into a particular area.

With the tools we have introduced so far, we can appreciate the relationship between movement strategies and anatomy. Bringing this knowledge together significantly increases the movement repertoire we can use with clients as they exercise. The exercises below will demonstrate the relationship between everyday movement and anatomy to further build that mind map of connections between the two.

By understanding movement before we apply it to anatomy, we can avoid most of the common restrictions and guidelines given to movement instructors. I am sure you have heard them—"the knee must not go beyond the toes," "the knee should always stay in line with the second toe," "when you do this exercise always make sure you bend/don't bend your spine." There are a few good reasons for these guidelines in group classes, as they are easy to follow, most people are familiar with them, and they can help the instructor keep everyone on track and safe. The problem comes when we start to apply those rules outside of classes and think of them as "rules for life." These rules are rarely necessary beyond the movement studio and could, in fact, be reducing our capacity for normal movement rather than increasing it.

Think about it—do you always want your knee to move straight over your second toe, or to never travel beyond the limits of your foot? How many different strategies do you use to bend and lift things when shopping or playing on the floor with your kids? We should work to increase the ranges and variety of movement and provide even more movement options for ourselves and our clients to ensure we can all continue to get on the floor and play with our grandchildren. Children at play do not follow the rules—and nor should we.

The hips and low back are probably the most complained about areas as people age.[4] Low back pain causes numerous lost days of work, and hip replacements are commonplace. One of the main reasons both areas become challenged is through lack of use. Limiting movement into an area will not only cause a reduction in strength but may continue to further reduce the ranges of motion used on a day-to-day basis. The solution is therefore for us to use the joints and keep challenging our clients' capacity to handle range and load.

Before we go further into an exploration around the hip joint, let's explore a quick exercise to get us warmed up. Stand up and perform a lunge to your right—step directly to the side with your right leg and keep your left leg straight (figure 6.9). Feel what happens in your left hip joint and where you feel a "stretch."

Now repeat the same exercise but this time step a little further in front of your first lunge. For example, if the first side step went to 3 o'clock, step to 2 o'clock this time (figure 6.10). Then repeat to 1 o'clock and finally to 12 o'clock. Where did you feel the reaction in the left hip?

If this was a suitable exercise for you, you most likely felt the change in the line of strain on the left thigh from very medial at 3 o'clock, gradually working its way to the front of the left hip when you stepped straight ahead at 12 o'clock.[5] There may or may not have been a surprise in that for you—the purpose of the exercise is to expose the relationship between movement direction and tissue reaction.

---

[4] Along with their false teeth, bladder problems, the state of the economy, their marriage, their kids never calling, and how you can never find a parking spot when you need one. But we can leave those for another book.

---

[5] Or it might have changed to the calf for the reasons we explored earlier.

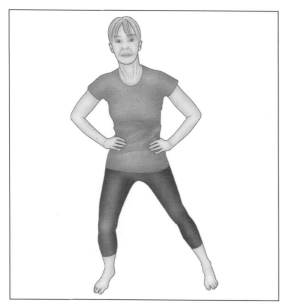

Figure 6.9. Perform a right side lunge by stepping to the side with and bending your right leg, keeping your left leg straight. Where do you feel a stretch around your left hip?

Let's take a close look at the relationship of the tissues around the left hip in figure 6.11 to see how we can start bringing some of our themes together. The ball-and-socket arrangement of the hip joint allows for a 360° range (though not equal in all directions), so each possible direction of movement must be matched by muscle tissue to provide support and control. As an aide-mémoire—everything in front of the hip is a flexor, everything behind is an extensor, crossing the outside are abductors, and crossing the inside are adductors—which helps us visualize the reaction in the tissues as the left hip responds to the movement of the right foot.

Learning to view muscles this way—by their position rather than by their named

actions—arms you with greater flexibility to interpret muscle action during movement. A common mistake is to revert to rote-learned "actions" when trying to comprehend soft-tissue performance during complex movement, but that often confuses as much as it enlightens.

We can continue the movement exploration further by taking the right foot to other points of the clock, to 4 o'clock, then 5, and 6 (figure 6.12). Of course, you don't have to limit yourself to the numbers on the face of the clock as there are many divisions in between the primary numbers. The movement could be fine-tuned by exploring the difference of just one or two degrees.

This simple lunge pattern around half the clock face might be enough for some people to "feel the stretch" on the stance leg and the "feel the burn" on the stepping leg as it does most of the work. However, we might need to adapt the exercise to make the stretches "stretchier" and the lunges more or less hard work. We will explore some ways to do that later, but first I recommend you try the same lunge pattern on the other side.

This time step out with the left foot and feel the reaction on the right hip as you keep it straight and let the right ankle adapt to the movement. You will be stepping to the other side of the clock (9, 10, 11, 12, 9, 8, 7, and 6) but it will be the same adductor tissues that you felt in the previous exercise (figure 6.13).

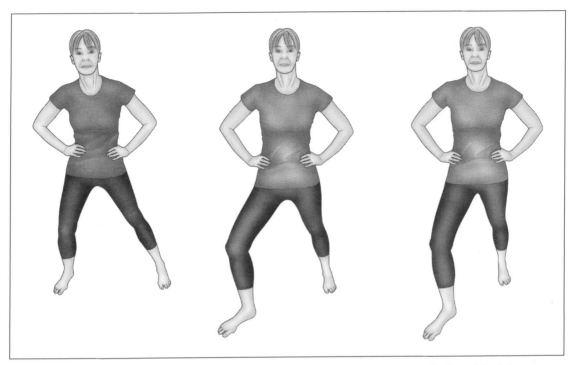

Figure 6.10. Repeat the side lunges working from 3 (figure 6.9) to 2 and then 1 o'clock, and feel the difference (if any) in the reaction at the left hip.

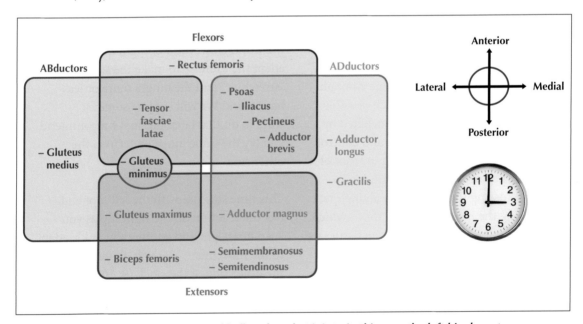

Figure 6.11. Tissue arrangements around ball-and-socket joints, in this case the left hip, have to cover every movement possibility. There is considerable overlap in the functions of the muscles, even though they are often grouped together as flexors, extensors, abductors and adductors. What is important, and what determines a muscle's reaction, is the angle at which it crosses the joint. Copyright Emma Armitage, 2023.

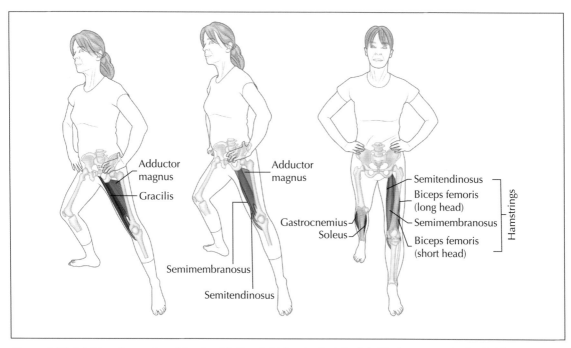

Figure 6.12. (a) Stepping out and back with the right leg to 4 o'clock is likely to stretch the "adductor extensor," adductor magnus of the left leg. (b) Stepping to 5 o'clock brings the stretch a little further round toward the medial hamstrings, the semimembranosus and semitendinosus of the left thigh. (c) Stepping straight back toward 6 o'clock brings us into an almost classic hamstring and calf stretch position.

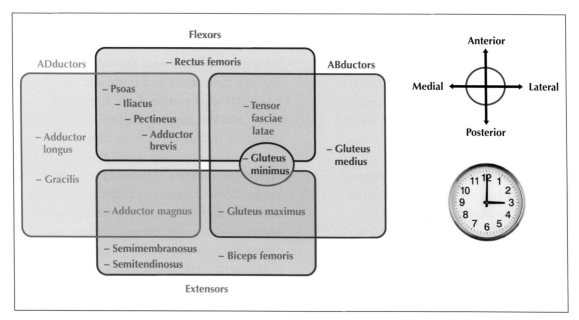

Figure 6.13. The tissue arrangement around the right hip mirrors that of the left. When seeing movement— or even when we prescribe it—we can think of targeting tissue groups or trying to improve the movement capacity in that area as it is impossible to isolate individual tissues. Copyright Emma Armitage, 2023.

Doubling Down by Bringing the Arms Up

You might not have felt particularly stretched or challenged by the side lunges above. That could be because you didn't push yourself and took small steps, or because you have adequate range of motion around the hip adductors. We can increase the demand for hip movement by also moving your hands as you lunge.

The possibilities are almost endless—one hand, two hands, same direction, opposite directions, higher or lower hand reaches … as you step out to the side, before you step, after you step … and so on. For now, we will confine ourselves to the target tissues of the adductors to further embed the power of what we can achieve through movement.

There is an interesting dynamic, an apparent paradox, in how we drive movement into the hip. Have a quick look back at the sagittal plane movements performed in the last chapter (figure 6.14). Taking the arms backward, up, and over the head created a demand for hip extension, but so too did taking the other knee forward.

The permutations for human movement probably outnumber those of a Rubik's cube, and would take just as long to explore. The keys to success are to take your time and regard the exploration as playful and open-ended. Keep in mind that, despite what the books might say, there are few definitive answers on how people move. Not everyone will perform the movements in the same way, there are always new and interesting interpretations to each exercise, and we must be happy in the place of not knowing. There are few absolutes in this journey, and this is just a guidebook to help clear some of the paths—but those paths keep splitting and dividing, splintering, and fragmenting. Looking for the unexplored avenues and cutting new tracks is all part of the fun of getting to know the human body.

Keeping those possible variations in mind, try the lunge variations with the same-side arm traveling overhead to the point on the clock opposite to the stepping leg (figure 6.15)—if the right foot goes toward 3 o'clock, the right arm goes to 9; if the right foot goes to 1 o'clock, the right arm goes toward 7.

You might need to experiment a few times to feel how far to reach with your hand to increase the sensation in the left hip. Or you might feel the reaction somewhere else in your system as you are now sending movement through your shoulder complex and into your trunk and spine, and that might be exactly what you need. Or it might be too much, and the stepping might be enough for you at the moment. Working with a friend can be informative and useful at this point to explore the differences between you. What works for one person might not work for the other, and exploring your differences builds experience in cueing for more or less range during the movements. Do not be afraid of asking for variation and exploring what happens—it is through experimentation that you will find your greatest moments of learning.

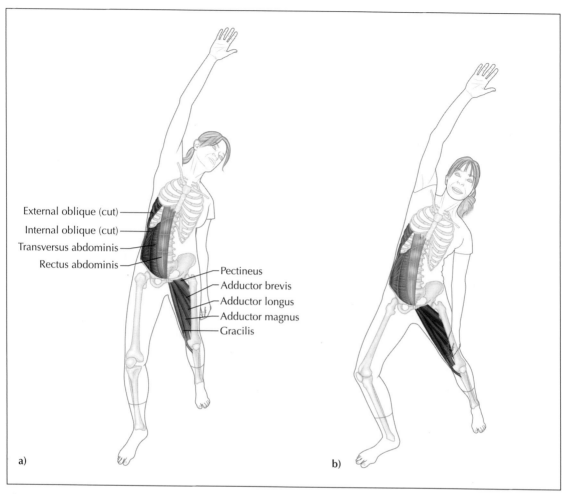

External oblique (cut)
Internal oblique (cut)
Transversus abdominis
Rectus abdominis
Pectineus
Adductor brevis
Adductor longus
Adductor magnus
Gracilis

a)

b)

Figure 6.14. Compare the reaction at the hip between the two side lunges, one to 1 o'clock (a) and one 2 o'clock (b)—left hip extension is increased by the right arm going backward overhead (a) and abduction is increased by the right arm coming across and overhead (b).

For example, try passing your hand across in front of the body as you step out to the side (figure 6.16), and contrast the reactions in the left hip. Experiment with the distance of the step and the reach. Alternate with the previous arm reaches, and notice the changes in your left hip and elsewhere. What do you think causes the differences?

Timing and Sequencing

The value of actions lies in their timing.
—**Lao Tzu,** *Tao Te Ching*

The trunk and pelvis (and therefore the spine and hip joints), are all affected by the movement of the arms. Compare the position of the rib cage between figures 6.14

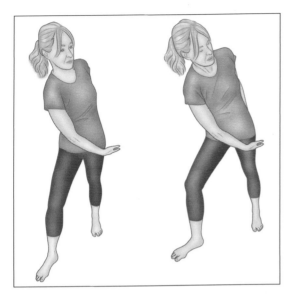

Figure 6.15. Perform the same side lunges as in figure 6.14 but bring your right hand across in front of your body. Contrast the two strategies by alternating between the arm passing up overhead and down and across in front—what difference does it make to the reaction at the left hip?

and 6.15—essentially, the trunk follows the angle of the arm and the tilt of the trunk will either increase or decrease the abduction of the standing leg. These movements can be adjusted in their timing—feel the difference between stepping out to 3 o'clock as far you can before reaching overhead and reaching overhead before stepping out to 3 o'clock (figure 6.16).

Not everyone will feel the effects of the variations above—reactions may depend on one's tissue type or the movement strategy—but they are useful experiments to play with as they reveal the movement relationships and interdependencies between our upper and lower bodies. Even the division—upper and lower—is arbitrary. Perhaps we should consider

movement references as differences between movement above or below the center of gravity. However you wish to think of it, being aware of the relationships and how they can affect one another can be incredibly useful for interpreting movement or creating personalized movement sequences for clients.

Simple examples of how one could combine the variables we have explored so far would be to:

- Side lunge with arm going overhead simultaneously: This should be a moderate-effort lunge.
- Side lunge without arm movement: This should increase the depth and range of the lunge to increase the load on the legs.
- Overhead reach of the arm and then side lunge: This will reduce the range of the lunge and therefore reduce the workload, and pretensioning some of the soft tissues will assist with the return.

Familiarity with the relationships between upper and lower body movement, timing, direction, and range will significantly improve how you see people move, especially in many sports.

Adding in the Abductors

Stepping out to the side with one foot created some degree of stretch to the adductors on the inside of the stance thigh. Now we need to bring balance to the outer portion of the "hip clock" and ensure we have enough range and strength in the abductors.

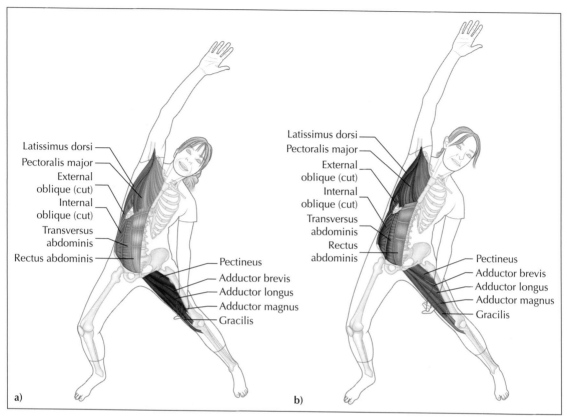

Latissimus dorsi
Pectoralis major
External oblique (cut)
Internal oblique (cut)
Transversus abdominis
Rectus abdominis

Latissimus dorsi
Pectoralis major
External oblique (cut)
Internal oblique (cut)
Transversus abdominis
Rectus abdominis

Pectineus
Adductor brevis
Adductor longus
Adductor magnus
Gracilis

Pectineus
Adductor brevis
Adductor longus
Adductor magnus
Gracilis

a)

b)

Figure 6.16. Sequencing can alter the reaction through the body. (a) Side lunging to end of range before reaching overhead is likely to reduce movement through the upper body and focus more strain into the adductors. (b) Reaching the arm across before side lunging might reduce the range of the lunge and make it more stable for some people.

Abductor stretches are most often performed in an open chain, allowing the leg to move in and across toward the midline (figure 6.17). Some people might claim that this is not a "functional stretch," but it might be exactly what is needed before executing more complex or stronger movements, and we should just quit the judging.

Another way to assess and to increase the capacity of the abductors is to drive the hip into adduction while standing. The easiest way to do this is by bringing the opposite foot across the midline in front and behind the standing leg (figure 6.18). Unlike the previous exploration of the adductors, where we could use a wide range (from 1 to 5 o'clock), this exercise achieves best results within a narrower band—say, 8 to 10 o'clock if reaching with the right leg.[6]

It is tempting to try to be precise as to which fibers of which muscles are doing the work,

_____

[6] If you wish to use the left leg, then the range is 2 to 4 o'clock.

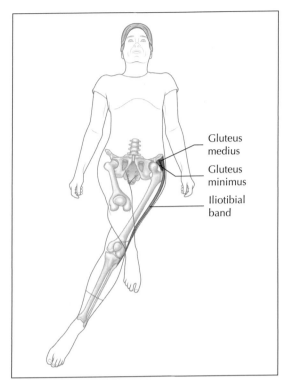

Figure 6.17. The easiest way for most people to stretch the abductors is to bring the hip into passive adduction.

but, once again, that is driven by textbook anatomy. Even in the adductor stretches above, we cannot really be sure that we are targeting any particular tissue. What we are doing is using movement to stimulate the area and increase the capacity for that movement. We can try to map it as best as we can to the muscle charts, but the soft-tissue reactions are complex and not always predictable.

That lack of predictability should provide encouragement to play with other variables, such as timing and the use of arm movements. From our experiments above we know that the upper limb can increase or decrease the range of motion at the hip during these movements. We can fine-tune the reaction at the hip to add

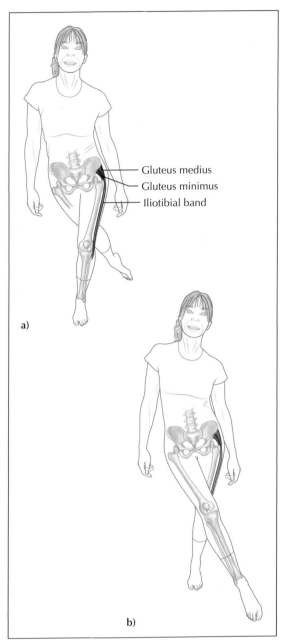

Figure 6.18. (a) Bringing the right foot across to 8 o'clock will adduct the left hip to bring strain into the gluteal area. (b) Changing the reach of the foot to 10 o'clock alters the flexion/extension angle of the hip and stimulates a different portion of the gluteals.

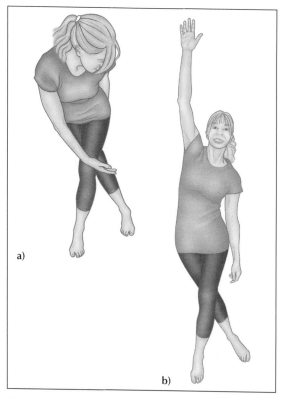

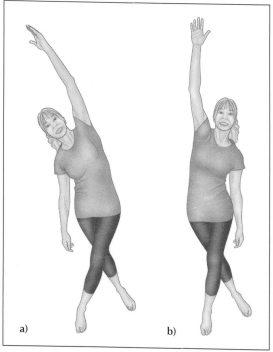

Figure 6.19. (a) Bringing the arm across in front of the body tends to tilt the trunk in the same direction as the pelvis and adds extra demand for adduction on the standing hip. Beware—this exercise can also challenge the standing knee. (b) The challenge to the knee, hip, and the abductors can usually be reduced by having the opposite arm elevated and even reaching across overhead. The right arm position and movement helps tilt the trunk in the opposite direction to the pelvis and tensions the tissue attachments along the top of the pelvis on the right.

Figure 6.20. (a) Bringing the left arm overhead as the right foot moves across to 10 o'clock increases the reaction toward hip adduction as it causes the pelvis and trunk to tilt in the same direction. This position can be unstable and may require some support for the right hand to hold. (b) Stability can be regained for the movement by raising the right arm, but this is likely to reduce adduction of the left hip.

extra load or to reduce it and make it easier. For example, having the leg and arm reach down and across at the same angle will increase the demand for adduction on the standing leg. In figure 6.19a, look at how the arm movement encourages the trunk to tilt along with the pelvis, which is following the right leg. Now contrast that to the elevated arm, which tilts the trunk toward the standing leg, in the opposite direction to the tilt of the pelvis (figure 6.19b). The elevated arm will also tension the tissue along the top of the pelvis on the right and help it decelerate as it drops away and, probably, reduce the overall range of movement.

To further build your body and movement map, I recommend trying the same movement with the right leg while using the left arm (figure 6.20). During this movement, the left arm passing overhead can increase adduction of the left hip because the shoulder complex causes the trunk to tilt in the same direction as the pelvis.

What we have learned so far:

- Lower and upper body drivers often cause opposite effects at the hip.
- The trunk responds to the direction of movement coming up from the pelvis and, more directly, to movement coming down from the arms.
- We can therefore use the arms to increase or decrease the reaction at the hip by moving them in ways that tilt the trunk in the same or opposite direction to the pelvis.

Summary

Our frontal plane explorations differ from those in the sagittal plane. The limitations of the hinge-like joints for flexion and extension contrast with the important ball-and-socket joints of the hip and shoulder. Although we did not break down the glenohumeral joint in the detail we used for the hip, the same principles can be applied to reinforce the relationships between muscle anatomy, joint architecture, and movement potentials. The rubric of "flexors in front, extensors at the back, abductors over the top, adductors crossing below, medial and lateral rotators crossing in front and behind respectively" is probably one of my most useful breakthroughs to help me *see* anatomy in action.

The principle of *range of movement*, the way we move in the real world, contrasts with the

range of motion we see in assessment manuals. Normal life requires numerous series of tissues during movement, and each joint between any fixed point and the target should make a contribution toward that goal. Our bodies are goal-oriented and will often sacrifice the comfort and integrity of an area to compensate for any functional loss along the movement chain. Each complex movement therefore has a series of *essential events* that can be analyzed and assessed to ensure they are responding appropriately.

If an area of the body appears to be withholding, we can start to implement the tools of positioning, drivers, and driver directions to encourage movement toward the misbehaving tissue. The therapist can choose to send movement into the body upward or downward by cueing the upper or lower body first.

When arm direction causes the trunk to tilt in the opposite direction from the pelvis, it increases lumbar side flexion, which may reduce the ability to move the hips into abduction or adduction—especially if the arm reaches across at the beginning of the movement.

Similarly, if the hips abduct or adduct first, there will be less range available for the arm movement. Unless the arm and trunk are moving in the same direction as the pelvis, in which case there is almost no lumbar flexion and hip movement will not be reduced by any limitation in the lumbars.

Some control of depth can also be achieved using the superficial shoulder girdle tissues. By cueing upper limb movements, the skin, adipose layers, pectorals, and latissimus dorsi can all have some degree of pretension that can help support the client. A possible side effect is that the superficial tension is likely to shield the deeper tissue from stimulation. Putting strain into the deeper tissues may require positions that also cause more instability owing to the lack of pretension around them.

Our bag of tools keeps expanding, and it is important to practice the vocabulary and the concepts to master their use. Although you might be tempted to jump ahead into the fun and excitement of the transverse plane, work through the exercises and questions below before moving on.

Reflection Questions

There are many things to think about from this chapter—revisit the discussions regarding the coupling between hip adduction, opposite side abduction, and low back side flexion.

1. How do you think that relates to the experiences you had during the movements shown in figures 6.15 to 6.20?
2. Consider the effects created by the direction of the arm movement and how it related to pelvic tilt.
3. What effect do you think the order of movement had on the ranges?

Think about what happens if you reach the arm at the beginning or the end of the movement.

4. What are the differences between *range of movement* and *range of motion*?
5. Choose a simple movement and break it down into *essential events*. What should happen at each joint and tissue? It can be useful to first ask what is the overall range of movement and which ranges of motion can be used to achieve it.

Notes

Limited space means that we cannot fully explore all the reactions through the body. One area that is worthy of extra attention is the foot and ankle complex, as it must manage the changes in the center of gravity as the body moves above.

For example, the talar joint is predominately oriented in the sagittal plane and manages the flexion/extension reactions, while the subtalar joint takes care of most frontal plane reactions through inverting and everting. Feel the different reactions through the ankle area when you step forward and back (figures 5.3 and 5.8) or side to side (figure 6.3). We will then compare these reactions with the rotations when we get into the transverse plane (chapter 7).

Twist and Shout

Shake it up, baby;
Now twist and shout.
Shake it, shake it up, baby;
C'mon and work it on out.

You know you move real good,
You know you move real fine.
—Phil Medley and Bert Berns,
"Twist and Shout"

The Transverse Plane

The transverse plane is the plane most movement teachers get excited about, and, as we will see, there are many good reasons for that. But I think it's a shame that our first two planes of movement are not given the same amount of attention, as they both have qualities that make us human.

Each species has its own unique movement strategies, which came about through a complex interplay between its ecology and its evolutionary and genetic history. As members of the primate family, humans developed movement patterns that evolved

from creatures that spent a lot of time in the trees. However—unlike the rest of the primate family—we developed the ability to stand upright and take long strides. Each long step requires stabilization along the outside of the stance leg, a uniquely human feature that assists with several energy-saving mechanisms within the myofascial system—a fact that is highlighted when we compare our locomotor costs to those of our close relative, the chimpanzee (figure 7.1).

If we were to break the planes down into simple features (something I normally resist doing owing to the risk of oversimplifying), our sagittal plane flexions and extensions provide us with range, and our frontal plane anatomy—especially the arrangement around the pelvis and thigh—provides the stability to stand on one leg as the other swings forward. And, if we continue along this reductive path, the transverse plane appears to provide us with power—the reason I and so many movement teachers get excited by it.

One reason why we should pay more attention to the sagittal and frontal planes first is that

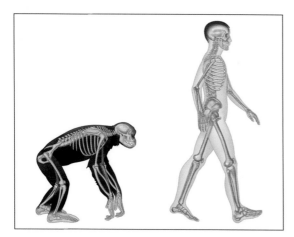

Figure 7.1. An upright stance with lateral stability provides the conditions for the long, straight-legged stride of the modern human. Reducing the number and the degree of bends at joints reduces the overall metabolic costs of walking and running and provides significant calorie savings.

we would find it more difficult to access the power of the transverse plane without them. To return to the examples of running and walking, it is our frontal plane stability that facilitates the longer stride, and the longer stride allows one lower limb to swing further than the other, bringing forth a rotation through the trunk.

That rotation takes advantage of the trunk's many obliquely oriented muscles, each of which is perfectly aligned to operate in rotation. The obliques, intercostals, deep spinal muscles, serratus muscles, pectorals, and latissimus dorsi (and many more) contain angled fibers. The various obliquely oriented muscles cross different joints at different degrees of depth. In doing so they provide joint control and connections between bones of varying degrees of separation, and thereby offer a wide variety of control and movement options.

Depth of Connection

Take a walk on the wild side.
—Lou Reed, "Walk on the Wild Side"

One of the many underexplored aspects of musculoskeletal anatomy is the general rule that deeper muscles cross fewer joints. There are notable exceptions in the hands and feet, but everywhere else the deepest muscle will cross just one joint to connect adjacent bones. The next muscle layer will probably cross two joints, the next will cross three joints, and so on. When one thinks about it, this arrangement makes sense. For example, placing the shoulder's one-joint rotator cuff muscles superficial to the multijoint trapezius would require perforations through the sheet of the trapezius for the rotator cuff to reach down to the scapula and humerus (figure 7.2).

As with most of our anatomy, there are evolutionary reasons for this organization. The development of the vertebral body was a series of adaptations that increased its complexity from a simple tube (let's call it the trunk, or thorax) to something much more complex with the addition of limbs (figure 7.3). Those limbs began with fins, which developed into the pectoral and pelvic girdles, and finally we also separated the head from the thorax by developing a relatively ribless cervical spine.

To maintain the integrity of the organs, which are safely protected within the trunk, each limb and the head developed on the body's outer layers. Our superficial muscles are therefore the youngest within our evolutionary story, and they are also the more

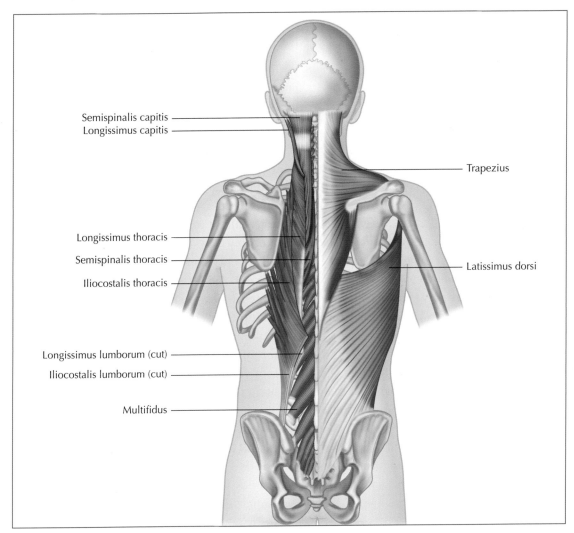

Figure 7.2. The logic of myofascial layers is rarely discussed in a way that reveals the relationships between position and function of the tissues. As a general rule, deeper muscles cross fewer joints. The deepest spinal muscles connect adjacent vertebrae. The next layer of muscle crosses two joints, then three, and so forth until we reach the longer fibers of the erector spinae group. The most superficial layer of the back, shown on the right of the diagram, illustrates how the trapezius and latissimus dorsi cross many joints and provide connection between the limbs. The trapezius connects the scapula to the head and to the opposite scapula (left trapezius not shown), while the latissimus dorsi is well known for its continuity to the thoracolumbar fascia and to the gluteus maximus on the opposite side.

complex in terms of angles and the numbers of joints crossed. The addition of each limb provided new and interesting locomotor potentials—potentials that were necessary for the changes from aquatic to terrestrial environment.

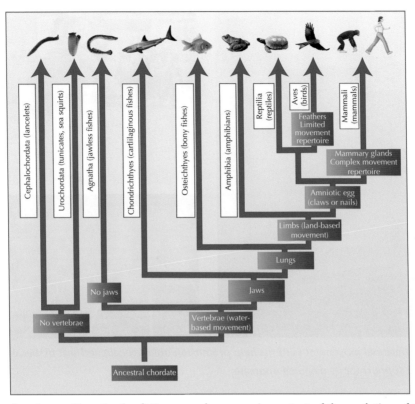

Figure 7.3. The layering and length of soft tissues makes sense in context of the evolution of the vertebrate body plan. Increased complexity in an animal's ecology is matched by increased complexity in its locomotor anatomy. Fins provided increased speed and maneuverability for avoiding predators and to catch prey but did not provide adequate stability for movement out of the water. Moving across the ground and working against gravity benefits from better-developed pelvic and shoulder girdles. The increased range of motion of the extremities benefits from the soft-tissue connections, such as the anterior and posterior oblique slings, running between them.

The anatomy of any animal makes sense only in the context of its environment. Body size, limb length, and joint ranges are all blended into an equation alongside climate, ecosystem, food sources, and the balance of predators and prey. It is ironic, therefore, that the species with possibly the widest movement repertoire has managed to create for itself an environment that limits the opportunities to exploit its movement potential.

That species is, of course, us. Humans do not excel at much. We are not the best swimmers, the fastest sprinters, the highest climbers or

jumpers. However, we can do almost everything. When we managed to combine that repertoire with tool creation and manipulation, our innate calorie-saving drive kicked in, with the result that we would rather sit in chairs than squat, drive cars than walk or run, and shoot guns (much too often) than throw sharpened sticks.

Complex movements such as swimming, running, climbing, and jumping benefit from long, multijoint muscles—the muscles that are most familiar to us. They are the first to be seen on the wall charts—pectoralis major, latissimus

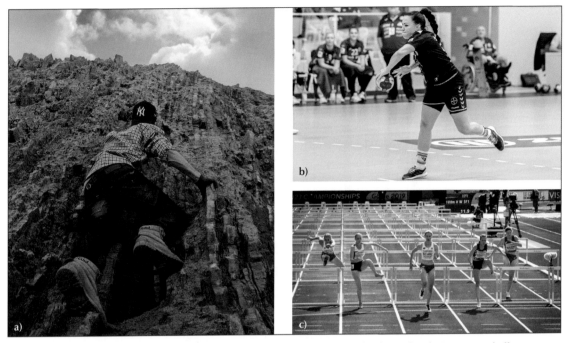

Figure 7.4. Contralateral movement patterns help pretension obliquely aligned soft tissues and allow one limb to provide support for its diagonal opposite.

dorsi, and trapezius, for example. But, as we explored in previous chapters, especially in chapter 1, we need to see movement to grasp the significance of the position of a muscle and the angles of its fibers. Movement provides the context for soft tissue, and, just as we need to see the wider ecosystem to understand the species, we need to explore beyond individual muscles to appreciate the true role of each muscle.

We have already seen that the contraction of a muscle can produce movement in joints beyond its attachments. The fact that movement of one area begets movement in another underpins functional anatomy and our tensegrity-based body, and most of those reactions do not require direct myofascial connection. For example, the abduction and adduction driven by the overhead frontal plane motion of the arms was a reaction of the whole body in relationship

with momentum and counterbalancing (see figure 6.3). However, some motions do take advantage of the myofascial continuities that connect the upper and lower limbs; recent research reviews have revealed strong evidence to support connections between our arms and thighs.[1] These connections between upper and lower limbs make perfect sense when we look at how we throw, climb, walk, and run (figure 7.4).

Soft-tissue pretension is automatically created through contralateral movement. Walking is the easiest movement with which to appreciate this dynamic—as one foot swings forward, the opposite hand also swings

[1]Jan Wilke, Frieder Krause, Lutz Vogt, and Winfried Banzer, "What Is Evidence-Based about Myofascial Chains: A Systematic Review," *Archives of Physical Medicine and Rehabilitation* 97, no. 3 (2016): 454–61.

forward. Both movements help to create pretension, as we will explore later. When our eyes start to see the overlap between the lines of tension created by the movement and the underlying, layered anatomy, we begin to see how this simple, everyday, and every-step action can pretension almost all the soft tissues through the trunk (figure 7.5).

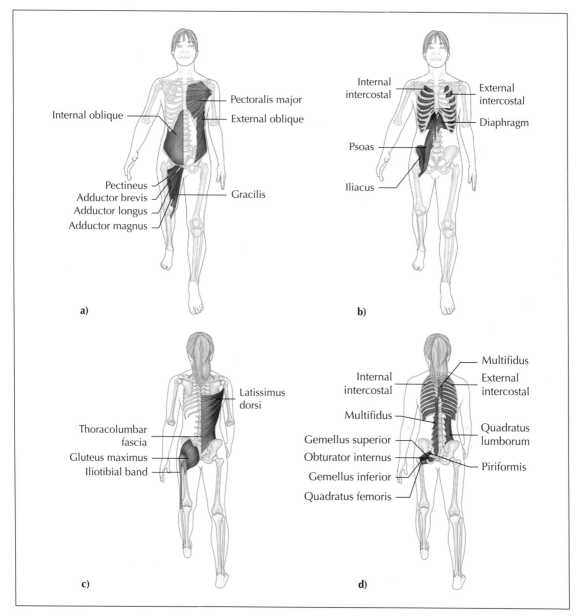

a)

b)

c)

d)

Figure 7.5. When we see the relationships at each joint, we begin to understand how our contralateral gait pattern creates pretension through many tissues. We can use the stabilizing superficial connections through the anterior and posterior oblique slings (or front and back functional lines of anatomy trains; a and c). By crossing fewer joints, deeper soft tissues provide more localized control to prevent the joints from collapsing, and by also pretensioning the deeper muscles can add significant force to the leg and arm swing (b and d).

Understanding pretension requires us to flip our heads away from the cognitive (learnt) bias of movement through "muscle action" and bones coming closer together. Bones also move apart to allow movement to happen—a fundamental element of what we have been exploring in this text so far—and as bones move apart, the connecting soft tissues must control that movement or the joint becomes unstable. Not only do the soft tissues help protect us from collapsing but in that lengthening we also recruit the benefits outlined in chapter 3:

- Possible capture of kinetic energy for recycling into the return movement
- Increased stiffness in the tissues, which can transfer energy more efficiently
- Working within the optimal force-length and force-velocity relationships.

Remember—most of our movements start by going in the opposite direction to pretension the soft tissues first.

Vocabulary Builder

Simply by changing your habitual vocabulary, you can instantaneously change how you think, how you feel, and how you live.

—**Anthony Robbins**, *Awaken the Giant Within*

Before we go further into the transverse plane and its many twists and turns, now is a good time to clarify how to describe movement. There is a well-developed language that, sadly, is not taught in most schools. I first learned the language 22 years into my practice as a therapist, and it made me angry. Not because of the words

that were being used, but because no one had ever taught me the difference between describing movement of a bone and movement at a joint.

There is a lot of looseness in movement and manual therapies over the words we use, but there doesn't have to be—in fact, there should not be.

To get a feel of the problem, what do you think people mean when they refer to the "hips?" Is it really the joint? Or the "hip bones?" If it refers to bones, which bones do they mean? Are your "hips" at the top of the ilia or at the width of the greater trochanters (figure 7.6)?

And what about the "knee"? Although there are fewer options here, what portion of the femur-tibia-patella interface are they referring to? And what would you do if I asked you to laterally rotate your right knee? Do you turn the patella to face laterally or turn the tibia laterally?

What about the frustrations of people's interpretation of "shoulder?" Is it the crest of the trapezius, the shoulder joint (if so, which one?), the shoulder girdle, or the whole shoulder complex?

We should also note that there is a *lot* of confusion about what constitutes the "shoulder," but there is a standard nomenclature for it:

Shoulder joint = the glenohumeral joint
Shoulder girdle = the scapula and clavicle
Shoulder complex = the scapula, clavicle, and the humerus

There are no bones or individual tissues called "knee," "hip," or "shoulder." These terms all relate to the relationships between bones—the joints. Of course, there are a lot of joint tissues between these bones, but there is no single

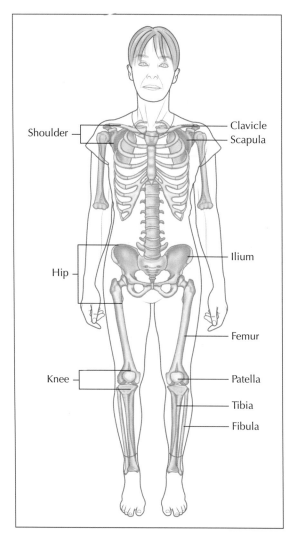

Figure 7.6. How we use the terms "hips," "knees," or "shoulders" in everyday life can depend on context. During normal conversation, the terms are defined by the ebb and flow of the conversation and often assisted by a lot of pointing. Confusion happens when we transfer that looseness into anatomy texts, which require precision.

There are no individual or specific structures labeled "hip," "knee," or "shoulder" on the right of the diagram. Each of those terms refers to the relationships between specific bones and should be used only in that context. In anatomy, the knee, hip, and shoulder are all joints and do not relate to any single structure.

structure called "knee," "elbow," or "hip." The names of joints are widely agreed conventions that—when used correctly in conjunction with movement descriptors (medial, lateral, abduct, adduct, etc.)—provide accurate images of what is happening in each joint-related tissue.

This may seem pedantic, but knowing how to describe the direction of bone movement and the resultant joint reactions is a major key in developing a visual understanding of four-dimensional anatomy. Take the example in figure 7.7. As the model turns to their right, there is a sequence of reasonably predictable reactions though the bones and joints—and we have to be clear with the language we use to describe them.

To perform the movement yourself, stand in a comfortable neutral with your feet roughly hip-width apart (i.e., the distance between the pelvis-femur joints). As you turn to the right, bring your awareness to your bones to feel how they react as you make the movement. Your pelvis turns to the right, as do the rest of the bones. However, your right and left femurs do turn to the right, but, for greater clarity, we must use the standard anatomical conventions:

- When describing movement of paired structures (such as femurs, tibias, humeri, etc.), we describe the movement in relation to anatomical position.
- When describing the movement of a single structure (such as the pelvis, thorax, or head), we use the cardinal terms of right, left, up, down.

This means that paired bones rotate medially or laterally, even though they might be rotating in the same overall direction. Although this might appear confusing when written down like this, I have no doubt you have already been

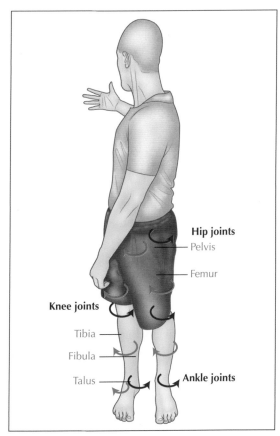

Hip joints

Pelvis

Femur

Knee joints

Tibia

Fibula

Talus

Ankle joints

Figure 7.7. Learning to describe bone movement and joint movement separately is key to "seeing anatomy in movement." It can take time to develop the necessary accuracy, but it is worth persevering with. We will build further detail onto this picture through the rest of this chapter and the next. For now, copy the movement shown by standing in a comfortable neutral position with your right hand lifted out in front of you. Look at your hand as you bring it around as far as is comfortable to the right. Allow your whole body to respond to the movement. Pause at the end of range and feel what has happened through your feet, knees, hips, and spine. Then bring your attention to the bones—the taluses, the tibias, femurs, pelvis, and spinal vertebrae as you move gently in and out of the position—can you feel the direction each bone moves as you turn to the right?

using this convention with ease, as we are all drilled in basic training on medial and lateral rotation of the hip and glenohumeral joints. It just gets a little less familiar when we realize that, as in figure 7.7, both femurs are turning in the same direction (to the right) but are described as medially and laterally rotating. We will see the reasoning behind this convention as we build the story in this chapter.

It is easy to become muddled when working with rotations—somehow it all gets twisted in our heads, and many of us struggle with left and right at the best of times, never mind when we are trying to interpret the written word alongside flat, two-dimensional images. I encourage you to do the movement outlined above, rotating in and out of the final position, to recheck what happens as you move.

It is important to keep in mind that you already use many of the verbal conventions smoothly without realizing it. Using right, left, up, and down to describe movement of the single structures is natural to us, they are the terms we use in everyday language, and they shouldn't cause us much stress. Everyone knows what is meant by the instructions to "turn your pelvis to the right" or "tilt your head up." It would make no sense to anyone if you asked them to turn their thorax, their head, or their pelvis medially or laterally.

How to Describe Joint Movement

Success and vocabulary go hand in hand. This has been proven so often that it no longer admits of argument.
—Wilfred Funk, *Six Weeks to Words of Power*

The way in which we define joint movement follows a couple of rarely clarified conventions. As bones on either side of the joint can be free to move in any direction at any time (within the constraints of their soft tissues), we need some form of agreement on how to describe what happens. Once again, this can seem like a lot of words, and they may appear to get in the way, but the conventions are in all likelihood the ones you are already using.

- Movement in the joints of the extremities is named according to the position of the distal bone (the one further from the center of the body). For example, if the femur is medially rotated in relation to the pelvis, the movement is described as "medial rotation of the hip."
- Movement in the spine is defined by the position of the superior vertebra relative to the vertebra below.

Naming spinal movement in terms of the superior vertebra provides continuity between everyday language and anatomy. It makes sense to us to "bend to the left" or "turn to the right" (figure 7.8). If movement in the spine was described using the same convention as for the extremities, a "bend to the right" outside anatomy class would turn out to be a "bend to the left" when we are in class.[2]

Thankfully there are no significant differences between the anatomical conventions and common usage, but many people do get confused when the bones and joints are moved in ways that differ from the standard muscle "actions." Let me reassure you that much of the confusion is not your fault. There are many books on exercise, Pilates, and yoga that are not consistent in their use of correct terminology. The antidote to continuing to make the same mistakes is to spend some time working through these few chapters. A thorough reading of this text will help you clearly visualize tissue reaction during movement, I promise.

Our goal is to become visually fluent with tissue reactions and to develop the skill of superimposing soft tissue anatomy onto the image in front of us. It does not matter whether the thorax moved away from the pelvis (figure 7.8a), or the pelvis moved away from the thorax (figure 7.8b and c), the line of tissue strain is the same—the same tissues will be lengthened and shortened (figure 7.9).[3]

Getting to the Core of the Matter

Vocabulary and its correct use are essential for describing and understanding anatomy. I know that might feel a bit scary, but it is really not that difficult, the main problem has been the lack of rigor in most training. The right rotation through the spine in figures 7.8 and 7.9 gives us the ideal opportunity to start peeling away some of the confusing layers that have held us back until now, as it gives us the opportunity to explore the important differences between describing the movement of bones and the movement of joints.

---

[2] I hope you have just bent to the right to work out why it would be a bend to the left if it were named for the position of the lower vertebra. It is because if the upper one is to the right, the lower one has to be to the left of the upper one. It will make more sense when you go back and read figure 7.8 and explore rotation. Trust me.

---

[3] Yes, of course, there will be some small differences because one movement might cause someone to extend or side flex more, but the overall tissue strain is the same. There's a time and place for absolute accuracy and pedantry, and this isn't it.

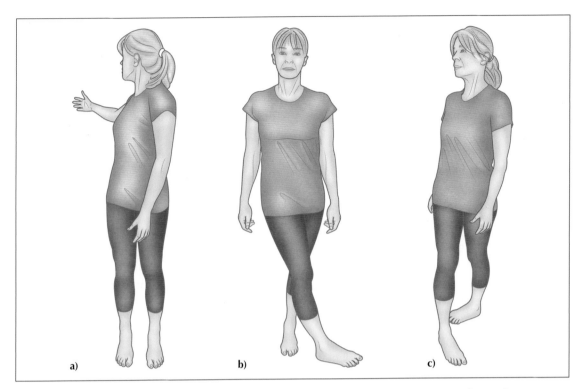

Figure 7.8. The convention for naming spinal movement according to the superior vertebra makes sense when we use it in everyday language. When performing the movement from the exercise above, we can clearly see how the spine will be rotating to the right to create a "right rotation of the spine." It becomes less clear when the spine reacts to movement coming up from the pelvis, as in the second movement (b). When the right leg steps around to the left, the pelvis also rotates to the left, as will each spinal vertebra, starting with L5, then L4, L3, and so on…

It is important to note that as we move up the spine, each vertebra is a little less rotated to the left than the one below it, and that means the spine has a right rotation passing through it, even though the individual vertebra may be traveling to the left. We can see the truth of this when we view the person from their front and compare the position of the thorax to that of the pelvis (c)—the thorax is to the right of the pelvis, the same relationship as shown in the first image (a). The implications of this are shown in figure 7.9.

This chapter has already emphasized the difference between joint and bone names and the traditions used to describe joint movement in the extremities or through the spine.

Movement of individual bones is referred to as "osteokinematics"—an apparently technical word but broken into its components a simple one to remember: we know *osteo* is anything related to bones, and *kinematics* is the study of movement. So, we are left with the obvious conclusion that *osteokinematics* relates to the movement of individual bones. But that does not always tell us what is happening at the joints.

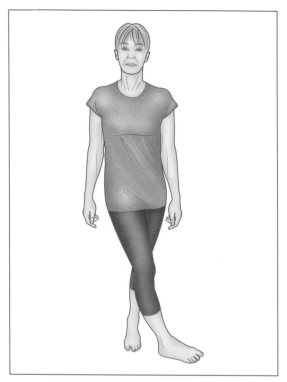

Figure 7.9. Right rotation of the spine causes the right external to left internal obliques to lengthen. It does not matter whether the thorax moves away from the pelvis or the pelvis moves away from the thorax (figure 7.8b), the line of strain remains the same. It is important to keep in mind, however, that how the tissues contract or change tone to create and control the movements will be quite different.

Movement at joints is referred to as "arthrokinematics." We already know the suffix *kinematics* relates to movement. The prefix is perhaps less obvious, until one thinks of the various conditions listed under "arthritis" (osteo-, rheumatoid-, psoriatic-), which all refer to pain and swelling in the joints. *Arthrokinematics* therefore refers to movement at the joints.

If this is the first time you have read about these terms you will be forgiven for wondering why I have given them so much build up, but, trust me, they are key to understanding tissue reactions and for creating new, precise, and specific movement interventions for you and your clients.

I have seen many movement teachers and therapists get confused by what you are about to read. If that happens to you, don't panic, just reread the next portion, look back to figures 7.8 and 7.9, and, most importantly, perform the movements in those illustrations for yourself.

Both movements in figures 7.8 and 7.9 created right rotation through the spine. The amount of rotation might not be the same throughout the spine, some portions may be more rotated than others, but the overall result was a right rotation of the trunk. We can see the implication of the movement by the lines of strain on figure 7.9, which illustrate the similar results in the tissues from the two movements.

Generally, people want to improve their hip flexion, their knee extension, or, as in this case, spinal rotation. We work to improve the relationship of bones at the end of the movement. I don't think I have ever heard of anyone asking to improve their femoral flexion, their scapular tilt, or their radial rotation. Our movement goals operate at the level of the joints and not individual bones, and if we want to improve hip flexion, knee extension, or spinal rotation, there are several strategies to help.

If we get stuck in the anatomical-model way of thinking, we will consider moving only the distal bones. For example, to improve hip flexion, the most common manual therapy strategy is to bring the femur up toward the pelvis while the client lies on the treatment table. However, as we have already seen, there are many ways to create movement through the body and they don't have to be driven by the target bone.

To return to the example of spinal rotation, we created right rotation of the spine by turning to right—a movement driven by the right upper limb. We also achieved right rotation of the spine by moving the right lower limb to the left. In these cases, the movement either trickled down into the spine from the upper limb or up into the spine from the lower limb. It is the second of those two movements, when the movement comes up into the spine, that often causes the confusion, as we rarely analyze the importance of direction (working through the examples in chapter 8 will help expand on these ideas).

Joint reaction is partly determined by the direction in which the movement travels into the joint. One easy way to categorize movement as it reaches the joint is whether it has traveled top-down (figure 7.8a) or bottom-up (figure 7.8b). So-called *top-down* directed movement comes from the superior bones moving further than those below, usually because the body part driving the movement is either the hands or the head. In contrast, *bottom-up* driven movement usually comes up through the body because of something we are doing with our feet or legs—stepping, kicking, running, squatting, or lunging. Each of these, if large enough, will cause the pelvis, the sacrum, and then the vertebrae to respond.

The Significance of Top-Down, Bottom-Up, and Joint Conventions

Now we see why conventions for naming joint movement (arthrokinematics) are important. Without the guidelines to follow, it would be easy to confuse the left rotation of the pelvis, which causes the lower spinal vertebrae to rotate to the left, as a "left rotation of the spine." The vertebrae certainly turned to the left, but the lower ones turned more than the upper, which means the spine is rotated to the right.

If the words get in the way, study figure 7.10 instead.

If this still does not make sense—and there is no judgment if it doesn't, as you are not alone in being confused by this—try the next exercise, shown in figures 7.11–7.13.

If you "get it" on one example, stick with that example—don't confuse yourself with others. If you have not "got it" yet, don't panic because we can use another example to help out.

Connecting with the Relations—Making Relationships Work

Interdependence is a higher value than independence.
—**Stephen Covey, *The 7 Habits of Highly Effective People Personal Workbook***

You will notice that the word "relative" is italicized in the last sentence of the legend of figure 7.13. That is because every joint is really a relationship between two, sometimes three

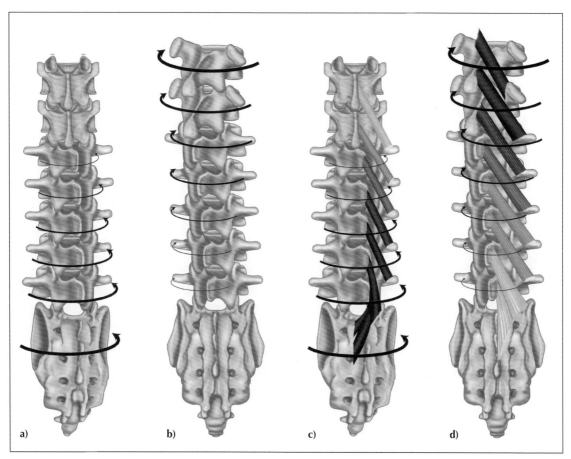

Figure 7.10. (a) As the pelvis turns to the left, movement comes up to the sacrum and to each of the lower vertebrae in turn. In this idealized example where the right foot is driving the movement and the rest of the body responds in sequence to it,[4] the lowermost bones will move most, with each bone above following in the same direction but moving less than the one below. This is referred to as "bottom-up" movement. (b) As the thorax and thoracic spine turn to the right, T11 and T12 will also turn to the right and each of the lumbar vertebrae will follow in the same direction, but the lower vertebrae will move less than those above. This is referred to as "top-down" movement. (c and d) Even though the sacrum and each vertebra rotated to the left, each superior vertebra was still "rotated" to the right of the one below. Rotation to the right causes the right lumbar multifidi to strain, and we see this pattern in both the bottom-up- and the top-down-driven rotations.

[4]This is an important point—the example used here is idealized. Real-life movement can incorporate numerous drivers acting simultaneously, which makes analysis much more interesting. These examples are just the first steps in getting familiar with the concepts and vocabulary.

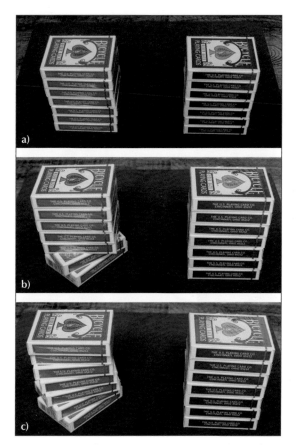

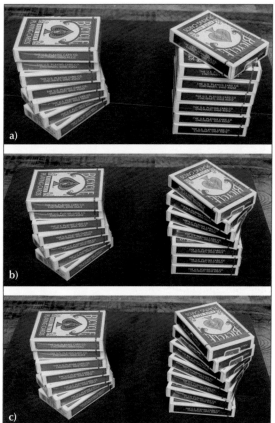

Figure 7.11. Collect as many square or rectangular objects as you can gather from around the house and divide them into two piles (drinks coasters are ideal, I just happened to have a lot of playing cards).[5] Use half of them for this exercise and reserve the others for the exercise in figure 7.12. Place the coasters (card boxes!) with one edge toward you (a). Consider the bottom coaster to be the sacrum and turn it almost one quarter to the left (b), then take the next coaster above the "sacrum" and turn it to the left, but a little less. Keep repeating the same action working upward through your pile, placing each one down a little less rotated to the left than the coaster below it (c).

Figure 7.12. Having created the stack of vertebrae rotated to the left, let's use the rest of the coasters and rotate them to the right. This time we start from above and give the top coaster a quarter turn to the right (a). We then work down the pile, turning each coaster below a little less to the right (b) to create a pile of coasters with each one turned to the right (c). Photographs for 7.11 to 7.13 courtesy of Michael Vincent.

---

[5]One could try this in a bar, where there is greater access to bar mats, but I recommend doing it early in the night as confusion can set in after the third or fourth drink.

bones, and the movement descriptors we use for joints are really describing the relationship between those bones. The only rule is that we name the relationship according to the conventions mentioned above—according to the distal bone for the extremities and according to the superior bone in the spine.

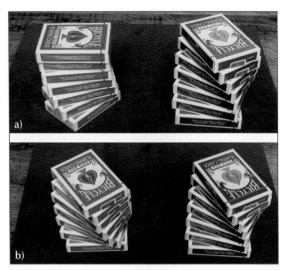

Figure 7.13. Place your two piles side by side, and they look quite different (a). If we bring the left-rotated sacrum back to neutral without disturbing the rest of the pile, we see that both piles match (b). The superior "vertebrae" are all rotated to the right relative to the ones below.

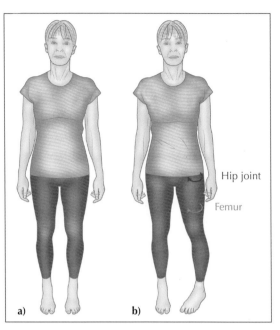

Figure 7.14. (a) Stand up, place your feet hip-width apart, and then (b) turn your left foot inward. What happened at your left hip? It medially rotated.

If the example in the spine did not make sense, then breathe easy, the example shown in figures 7.14 and 7.15 is simple.

As with the example of right rotation of the spine, the same tissues will be lengthened if we medially rotate the hip using a bottom-up- or top-down-driven movement.

BUT—different muscles will be involved in creating the movement. Too often we directly associate the joint movement with the relevant muscle actions, but that is not always the case. In figure 7.14, the medial rotation is mostly caused by the medial rotators of the hip, probably mostly tensor fasciae latae. In figure 7.15, the medial rotation of the left hip is mostly caused by the swing of the right leg, and the medial rotators of the left hip are quiet. During both movements, the lateral rotators

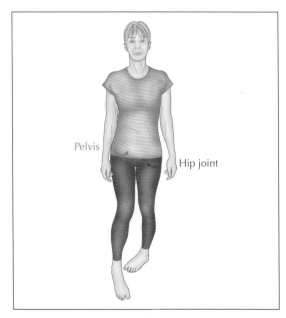

Figure 7.15. Now come back to the same position (figure 7.14a). This time, step around to the left with your right foot and let the rest of your body follow. What happened in your left hip this time? This movement also created medial rotation of the left hip.

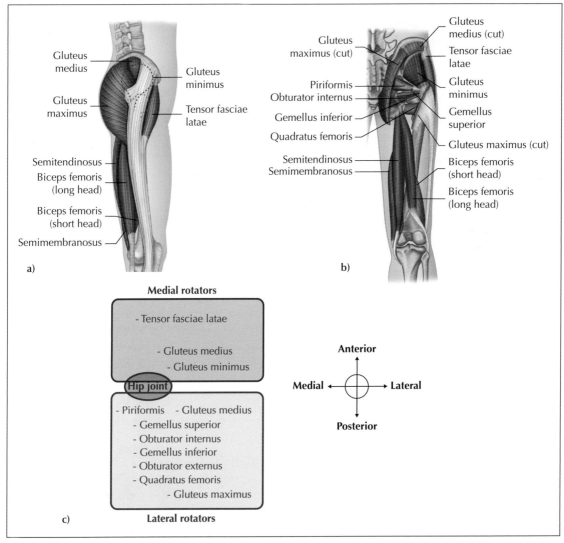

Figure 7.16. To create and control their wide movement range, ball-and-socket joints have muscles crossing them from every direction (a and b). Although this appears complicated at first, seeing the fiber angles and where they cross the joint provides us with most of the information we need to interpret muscle action. As explored in figures 6.11 and 6.13, flexors and extensors cross the front and the back of the joint respectively, while abductors cross the outside, and adductors are on the inside of the joint.

(c) Joint rotation is controlled by muscle fibers crossing at the joint at an angle. As a general rule, those crossing the front of the joint will medially rotate it (e.g., tensor fasciae latae) and those crossing the back of the joint (for example, all of the bundled lateral rotators of the hip) will laterally rotate it.

of the left hip will probably increase their tone to help control the movement as they lengthen.

Unlike the earlier exercise when the hip was flexed, the hamstring group will be less able to create hip rotation from the neutral position.

Their control of hip rotation increases when the ischial tuberosity moves posteriorly as the hip flexes (see figure 5.4).

Completing the Third Dimension of Ball-and-Socket Joints

I make music for the hips, not the head.
—**Fatboy Slim, IMDb biography**

If you were paying attention in chapter 6 you might have noticed that we covered only flexion/extension and abduction/adduction of the hip joint in figure 6.9. Now we should add the transverse plane to complete the picture.

As a reminder—muscles that cross the front of joints are flexors, and those that cross the back of joints are extensors (keeping in mind the in-utero twist of our lower limbs that brings the "front" to the back and vice versa). Any muscle that goes over the top of a ball-and-socket joint will help abduct it, while muscles crossing the inside of the joint will adduct it.

There may be slight variations and deviations from these general guidelines, but this rubric mostly hangs true and, I would argue, is a more flexible way to learn functional anatomy as it provides adaptability for interpretation when trying to analyze complex movement.

The final portion of the guidelines addresses the transverse plane—any muscle crossing the front of a joint at an oblique to horizontal angle will be a medial rotator; lateral rotators tend to cross the back of the joint at oblique or horizontal angles (figure 7.16).

Of course, there are a few muscles that do not fall into this neat "close to horizontal" pattern. For example, latissimus dorsi comes from the lower back all the way up under the arm to attach at the front of the humerus. Crossing to the front of the arm means that the lats can pull the humerus into medial rotation—an essential action for climbing and throwing. The lats are assisted in these actions by the teres major, which also comes from the back of the body, but from the scapula, to attach alongside the latissimus dorsi on the front of the humerus (figure 7.17).

There are a few muscles around the hip joint that pass from the front to the back, and these tend to be the ones with debated "actions." The psoas is probably the most famous of these, as references will list it

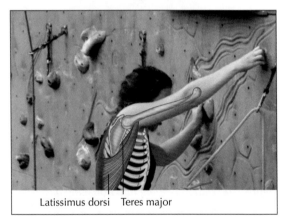

Latissimus dorsi   Teres major

Figure 7.17. The latissimus dorsi and teres major both pass under the glenohumeral joint to attach to the front of the humerus. Both muscles exert strong forces to assist medial rotation at the glenohumeral joint; however, they can also control the scapula (especially teres minor) and trunk (latissimus dorsi) to draw them toward the anchored supporting arm. This reversal of "action"—bringing the trunk toward the humerus—is key to appreciating the size and the myofascial connections of the latissimus dorsi.

variously as a medial or a lateral rotator of the hip joint. The confusion is caused by the way in which the psoas, along with the fibers of the iliacus, passes over the front of the ilium and then travels backward toward the lesser trochanter. My own bias is to suggest that psoas is more likely to laterally rotate the hip joint when standing in neutral. However, if the hip joint is abducted or flexed (or a combination of both), the iliopsoas tendon will not be traveling "backward" from the lip of the pelvis and could easily assist with medial rotation of the hip (figure 7.18).

The anterior adductors are another confusing group of hip muscles, as, like the psoas (which

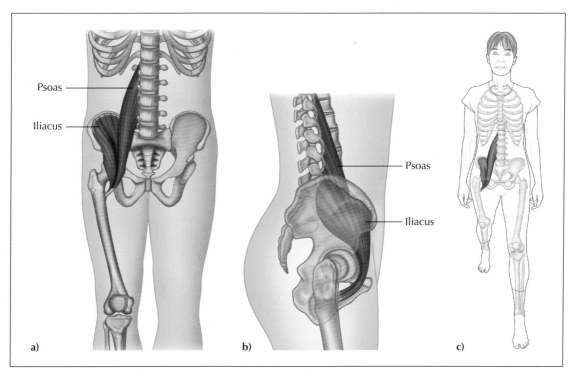

Psoas

Iliacus

Psoas

Iliacus

a) b) c)

Figure 7.18. Understanding functional myofascial anatomy relies on the ability to visualize how the muscles cross joints in any position. When a joint moves, the muscle-fiber angles will adjust accordingly and sometimes that will affect the possible "actions" a muscle can exert. In anatomical position, the conjoined iliopsoas tendon travels backward from the front of the pelvis to the lesser trochanter. This angle allows the psoas to assist with hip flexion and lateral rotation (a and b).[6] The angle at which the iliopsoas crosses the joint changes when the hip is flexed and abducted (c). In these positions it is possible for the tendon to exert a medial rotation force.

---

[6]Yes, I know the flexion action of the psoas is strongly debated in some anatomy nerd circles. I do not find the discussion to be enlightening, as most of it is based around action from anatomical position and therefore significantly limited in scope.

is also an adductor as it crosses the inside of the hip joint), they travel from the front of the pelvis to the back of the femur. For many years I assumed the linea aspera, the line of adductor attachment along the thigh bone, was medial on the femur. It was only during an advanced training that I realized the linea aspera is actually on the back of the bone, meaning the adductors have to wrap around the thigh to travel from front to back. This slightly unusual arrangement is another result of that in utero twist of the lower limbs, which also wound up the myofascial tissues and ligaments of the anterior hip. The twisted ligaments and joint capsule explain why humans are relatively limited in both hip extension and medial rotation at the hip joint (figure 7.19).

Let's take a moment to explore the implications of the hip's twisted ligaments and anterior adductors by coming back to the sagittal plane lunge (figure 7.20). When the lunge is performed according to the "rules," and the foot, knee, and hip are all aligned, most people will feel a "stretch" in the calf or at the front of the hip joint. If you feel the stretch in the calf, remember that you can reduce that by adding a wedge under the back foot to decrease ankle dorsiflexion.

Perform the lunge in at least three positions. Have your back foot pointing straight ahead to feel your "normal" reaction at your hip, and then repeat the lunge with your back foot turned inward and then turned outward. Most people will quickly sense the impact of lateral rotation freeing up more movement at your hip.

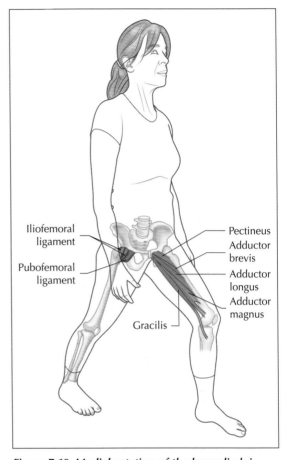

Figure 7.19. Medial rotation of the lower limb in utero causes many ventral tissues to wrap around the front of the hip joint and travel toward the back of the femur. The ligaments (shown on the right hip) follow the anterior adductors (pectineus, adductor brevis, and adductor longus, shown on the left hip) as they pass from the front of the body toward the back. We call our upright stance "neutral"—however, it is not really neutral for our hip joints. In anatomical position, the joints could be considered as extended and medially rotated. This prepositioning explains why we are limited in extension and medial rotation in comparison to other hip movements.

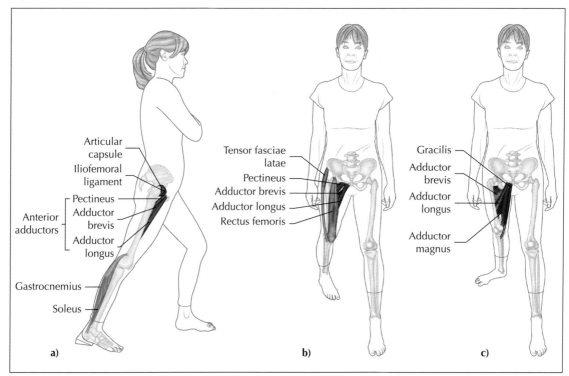

Figure 7.20. (a) An increased distance between the two feet to perform a lunge aligns the feet and knees of both lower limbs but will eventually cause the back hip to medially rotate slightly, as the pelvis turns toward that side and often causes more strain in the calf of the back limb. (b) Using a wedge to lift the back heel reduces ankle dorsiflexion and will allow more movement of the back hip. Experiment with longer and shorter lunges with your back foot turned inward. Which position allows you to rotate further inward? It will normally be when the back hip is less extended in the shorter lunge. (c) Do the same experiment with your back foot turned outward. What is the greatest change you notice?

Prepositioning and Fine-Tuning

I'm in a position that allows me to do what I want to do, and I do it.
—Eddie Murphy, FaceBook, March 5, 2014

The experiment in figure 7.20 that you just did is an introduction to the effects of prepositioning for exercise. Whether you practice yoga, Pilates, or functional exercise you can fine-tune the prepositioning to create certain effects.

Hopefully, you just felt how some stances increased the range of motion at the back hip and others reduced it. Increasing and decreasing motion are neither good nor bad—they are just reactions. In some cases, we might want to choose a position that allows the hip to move easily; in other situations, we might want more stability in that area. Now we can make an informed choice of positioning to help create the desired reactions.

Go back to some of the exercises in chapters 5 and 6 where upper limb movement is used in combination with different foot positions. How does each movement feel if you have more or less range at your hip owing to the hip's starting position?

Many movement teachers have been taught the "best way" to position the feet prior to beginning an exercise. Sometimes these "best ways" are historical, passed from guru to guru, and sometimes they were developed for the safety of group exercise. But the instructions became generalized into "good practice," regardless of client needs and individual differences. It is important to remember there are no good or bad exercises or positions, there is just *movement*, and we can adjust the many variables to find the best fit for our client's needs and safety using the many skills we have—prepositioning is one of those skills.

Prepositioning the feet is only one way of affecting movement. Try repeating the simple side bend in chapter 6 (figure 6.6) with two different strategies. First, reach up and across with your arm, and then reach the same-side leg across—feel the reaction. And then, reach across with your foot before bringing the same-side arm up.

> Do you feel a difference?
> Do you see a difference in the sequencing if you watch a partner perform the action?
> What is the difference in the spine? (Think bottom-up vs. top-down.)
> Is there a difference in the overall range of movement?
> Which joints are providing more or less range of motion?

Stable and Unstable Part 1: The Power of the Transverse Plane, across the Back

Stability is not immobility.
—**Klemens von Metternich, Congress of Vienna, 1814–15**

Finding positional sweet spots is a matter of trial and error if you are prescribing exercises, but you can also see the influences of prepositioning during everyday and sporting activities. We played with the effects of reduced ranges of motion earlier (figure 2.3)—by reducing the range of one joint we either force others along the chain to compensate by increasing their range or reduce the overall range of movement.

We like to distribute load through many tissues during long-chain movement. We take advantage of the many force-enhancing and dispersing qualities of the fascial tissues both locally, at each joint, and globally with direct and indirect myofascial relationships. Obviously, the significance of force distribution increases as forces increase, and, if we need more force output, we need either stronger, stiffer myofascia or to use more myofascial units. Some dynamics that affect force output are inherent within the architecture of the myofascia (tendon stiffness, fiber angulation, number of fibers, etc.), but these focus on the force production across the joints associated with the named myofascia, not necessarily the performance of the whole body.

To give a real-world example, I was asked to assess a UK Premier League soccer player.

At 17 he was still trying to break through to the senior squad but was hampered by what his physiotherapists referred to as a "weak glute" problem. The player had ruptured his anterior cruciate ligament twice—not something one wants to do in professional soccer.

All the squad had been videoed during a series of screening tests, including a shuttle run in which they were asked to run to a line, decelerate, turn, and run back to another line, and keep repeating the run until exhausted or out of time. The physical therapy department showed me their star performer first. This guy had "buns of steel"—he hit the line, decelerated smoothly, controlled his knee alignment, and took off again back to the other line (figure 7.21).

The player with "weak glutes" failed to perform the task with the same accuracy or efficiency and in particular struggled to control the limb he used during the deceleration and turn. The physical therapists all agreed there was a difference between the alignment of the players' supporting knees, and this was taken as proof that the player with the challenged ligaments needed to strengthen his glutes to better control his lower limbs. The problem was that no matter what he did in the gym, his test did not improve.

What the therapists were missing was the overall body positioning and deceleration strategy. Look at the difference in hand positions between the two players. Strong-glutes guy has his opposite hand in front of the loaded knee (figure 7.21a), while weak-glutes guy has his opposite hand above his head (figure 7.21b).

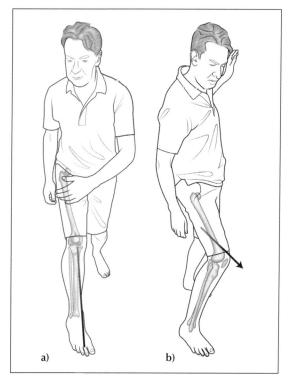

Figure 7.21. (a) "Buns of steel" guy runs to the line and decelerates. He can keep his knee over his second metatarsal, an indication of good control and strength in his glutes, as they control the flexion, adduction, and medial rotation at the hip to support the knee. (b) "Weak glutes" guy performs the same run but his knee drifts inside his second metatarsal when he decelerates, causing the knee to come into valgus, a dangerous position for the cruciate ligaments.

Now look carefully at the two positions. Strong-glutes guy has his loaded hip flexed, medially rotated, and adducted. Weak-glutes guy has his loaded hip flexed, slightly abducted, and less medially rotated, which is not a strong position for gluteus maximus. By bringing the hip into flexion, adduction, and medial rotation, the stronger player has pretensioned his gluteus maximus in each plane and has created strain along the iliotibial band (ITB). The pretension in gluteus maximus and the ITB both help prevent the knee from moving into valgus.

The weak-glutes guy has not achieved the same amount of pretension in his gluteus maximus or ITB, and his knee is able to migrate inward. But this was not because of any weakness in his glutes (remember he is in the gym every day, and if he is not in the gym, he is playing football!), it is because he did not put his hip into the same position of advantage as his teammate. Weak-glutes guy was not weak in his glutes, something was not optimal in his movement strategy. So, we looked at his arms.

It would be natural for most of us performing a shuttle-run test to run, hit the line, and decelerate with our opposite arm across our body, almost reaching toward the loaded knee. But weak-glutes guy's movement strategy was different. He preferred to take his opposite arm up over his head. We did some exercises in chapters 5 and 6 that showed what effect that can have—if we take the arm up and back (sagittal plane), the hip will extend, and if we take it out and over the head (frontal plane, abduction), the opposite hip will abduct. But during the deceleration phase of the shuttle run, we want the hip to medially rotate, flex, and adduct. The problem was not the guy's glutes, it was his overall movement strategy— he needed to move his opposite arm toward the loaded knee, not away from it.

Of course, it is not only the gluteus maximus controlling the knee during the deceleration. The hand and arm reaching around the body will also tension the tissue of the latissimus dorsi and the thoracolumbar fascia (TLF). This sequence of myofascial tissue—latissimus dorsi, TLF, to the opposite gluteus maximus

(GMax)—crops up in at least two well-known maps of continuities and is one of the few that stands up to investigation for consistency and ability to transfer force.

Named the *posterior oblique sling* by Dutch physiotherapist Andry Vleeming and the *back functional line* by Thomas Myers, this superficial layer of tissue connects the upper and lower limbs. It should be noted that the two analyses differ at the gluteus maximus: Vleeming uses the better-established connection between the TLF and superior GMax into the ITB, while Myers suggests taking the lower fibers of GMax and continuing into the vastus lateralis. The reality is that it does not matter—the body works as a whole—and this type of disagreement is quite academic. The likelihood is that both levels of connection, superior and inferior fibers of GMax, will tension to assist movement control.

The continuity from upper to lower girdles has many potential uses: increased power in sprinting, helping to control the body in landing, climbing, and helping to decelerate change of direction. Compare the two positions for our soccer players. The first one has consistent tension through the back line (figure 7.22a), while the hand position of the other has not only changed the local joint position around the hip but also shortened the sling (figure 7.22b).

While many therapists focus on the soft-tissue relationships and their continuity through the anterior and posterior oblique chains, it is also important to see the rhythm of movement through the skeletal system. Position yourself as in figure 7.22b, and then slowly allow your raised hand to come across and above your

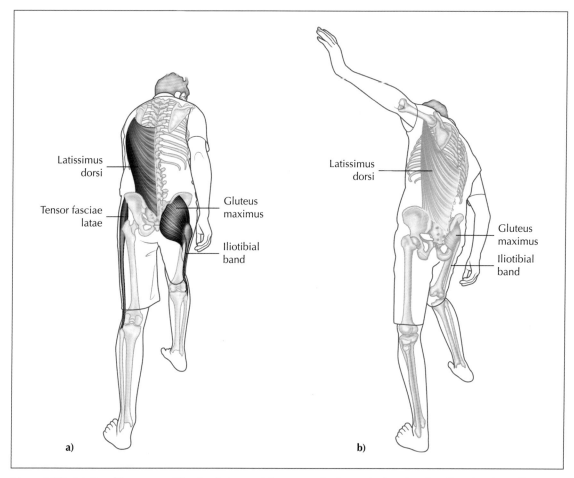

Figure 7.22. (a) Reaching around the body toward the opposite knee during deceleration tensions the myofascia from the gluteus maximus to the opposite latissimus dorsi. The pretension creates a sling of support for the relatively heavy pelvis, helping the gluteus maximus and ITB to decelerate the pelvis, control the knee, and change direction. (b) Using an alternative strategy with the opposite arm fails to load the posterior oblique sling in the same way, reducing its ability to provide force and control for the knee.

right knee. Let your body react and follow the movement—what happens to the valgus position of your forward knee? Did it correct naturally as a response to the movement of your hand? If not, try alternating between the two positions with a little more speed—did that make a difference? If it does not happen for you (which is about 10% of people, in my experience), try watching someone else perform the movement.

Most people will naturally correct the knee as the bones and joints through the trunk respond to the oblique movement of the upper limb. As the hand comes down and across, it causes the trunk to flex and rotate, which causes the forward hip to flex and adduct. As the hip adducts, the distal femur tends to move laterally and thereby corrects the valgus position.

In the case of weak-glutes guy, we could choose to discuss his myofascial continuity, his bony rhythm and coordination, or his development of motor control patterns. The truth is that they all overlap—the myofascial-skeletal patterns through the body's anatomy match our movement strategies, and our motor control development should optimize when our nervous system coordinates movement that takes advantage of the natural patterns within us.

Stable and Unstable Part 2: The Power of the Transverse Plane, across the Front

The stability we cannot find in the world, we must create within our own persons.

—Nathaniel Branden,
The Six Pillars of Self-Esteem

The physical therapists got more and more interested as we watched videos of the two players to analyze their different movement strategies, especially since weak-glutes guy had not only challenged his cruciate ligaments but also was prone to groin strain.

Thankfully, they had recorded a full battery of soccer-specific tests, one of which was kicking a ball. We started with "good guy" and saw him run up and strike the ball just as you would see on TV (figure 7.23a).[7] His left arm came out to the side and upward

as his right foot cocked back for the strike, and then he hit the ball sweetly and followed through with his opposite limbs coming forward (figure 7.23b)—a similar relationship to the one we saw in the deceleration above (figure 7.22a).

It is probably no surprise that "weak-glutes and groin strain" guy did not follow the same strategy. As he ran up to the ball, he also cocked his right leg back, but rather than the left arm coming up and back, it came forward and down (figure 7.24a). Failing to bring the arm up and back was reducing the pretension in his superficial tissues and putting all the kicking force into his local hip flexors, probably causing tissue overload.

The follow-through looked equally uncomfortable. Even though the arm was forward, it was held so tightly to his side that it contributed little to tissue tensioning or deceleration of the kicking leg. The conclusion we came to was that this guy had not developed good contralateral movement patterns. He did not need to strengthen any particular tissue, he needed to improve his motor control strategies. We suggested trying various cross-crawl-type exercises—anything that would help practice opposite limb relationships.

Stable and Unstable Part 3: The Power of the Transverse Plane, through the Layers

I think the golf swing is all about rotation, all about trying to keep the club on plane.

—Tiger Woods, *Golf Digest*,
January 2005

---

[7]If you had the time and patience to watch soccer on TV, but you will see the same shape when passing any ball-kicking game in the park.

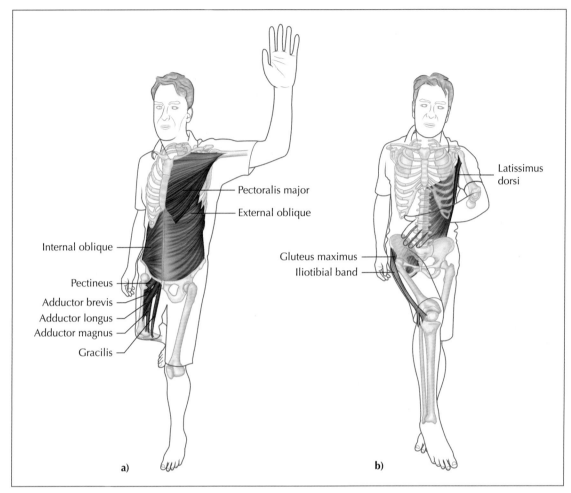

Figure 7.23. (a) During the run-up, the player prepares for a powerful kick by reaching his arm out to the side while the opposite hip cocks back into extension and abduction. This contralateral pattern pretensions the superficial myofascia on the front of the body from the upper to opposite lower limb using the many obliquely oriented tissues. (b) The deceleration of the kicking leg occurs during the follow-through after the kick and is assisted by tensioning across the back in a similar pattern to that used during the shuttle run (figure 7.22a).

As with the posterior sling, there are different versions of the anterior contralateral continuity. Myers suggests the pectoralis major to the rectus abdominis to the opposite adductor longus, while Vleeming uses the external and internal obliques to the opposite anterior adductors. As with the posterior slings, some of the discussion is academic rather than practical—the reality is the body uses the tissues whose angulation of fibers matches the orientation of the movement. A more vertical, sagittal reach of the upper limb will use the rectus abdominis, while a more transverse plane one will recruit the angled fibers of the obliques.

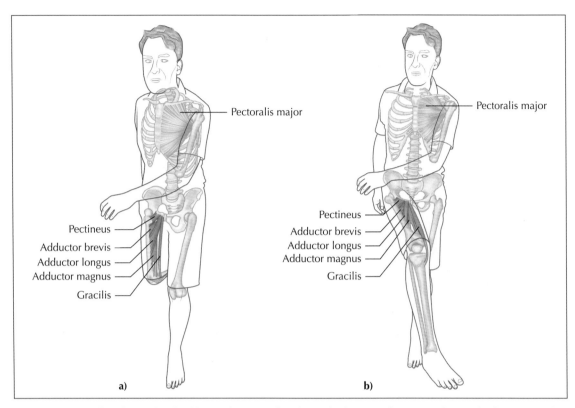

Figure 7.24. (a) The player that had been diagnosed with weak glutes and a strained groin had an unusual kicking style. Rather than using the contralateral cocking to strain the anterior oblique sling and all the associated flexor and rotator tissues of the trunk he kept his opposite arm adducted. This movement strategy can be useful for soccer players during a game to prevent telegraphing a kick, and it also requires less preparation time. But its repeated use places more stress on the localized hip flexor tissues, as the superficial muscles joining the trunk and the shoulder girdle have not been pretensioned. (b) The player's adducted opposite arm did help with the deceleration and control of the follow-through and uses a similar strategy as explained above (figure 7.23). However, the adducted position of the upper limb fails to give the same degree of initial support as that achieved by his teammate's strategy.

The twist through the torso created by contralateral movement also affects the deeper myofascial layers of the trunk, the intercostals, and multifidi. The crisscross pattern of the internal and external intercostals means that, regardless of direction of turn, both sides of the trunk will be tensioned. These tissues can act like a watch spring, getting wound up in one direction before releasing energy to encourage a twist in the opposite (figure 7.25).

It's Deep, Man

The contralateral relationships explored above show the stabilizing and power-enhancing properties of the superficial connections between the upper and lower limbs, as well as the pattern in the deeper tissues that get wound up during rotational movement. We also noted that most of our tissues follow the model of superficial and long to

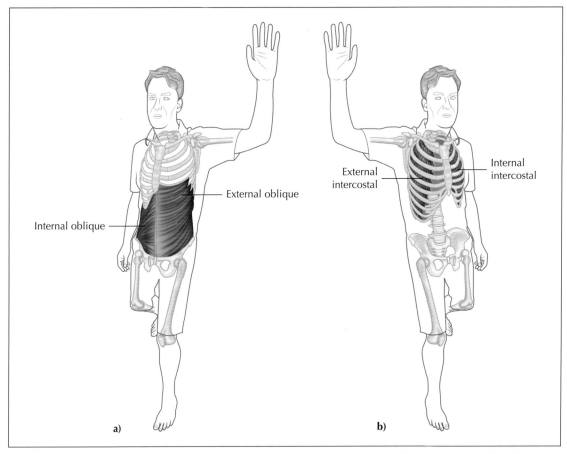

Figure 7.25. (a) According to fascial researcher Carla Stecco, the external and opposite internal obliques can be considered as one digastric (two-bellied) muscle connecting the lower ribs to the opposite side of the pelvis. This same angulation can be seen in the shorter external and internal intercostals, which also become tensioned during rotation. (b) The whole trunk can act like a watch spring as it tensions in either direction.

deeper and shorter. The areas in which that doesn't hold true are in the distal limbs— the forearm and hand and the leg and foot. Although not related so much to transverse plane movement, these exceptions are worth mentioning as they emphasize an important principle.

Primates need control of their distal phalanges, especially humans in our hands. Our fingertips do a lot of work, and they have to be not only dexterous but also able

to grip hard if, for instance, we need to hang on to a precipice. The phalanges are small bones that have to move a lot and produce a lot of force. We do not want short muscles attaching to them, as they won't offer the same controlled range of motion as muscles with longer fibers that can shorten and lengthen over greater distance. Nor do we want our hands and feet filled with bulky strong muscles capable of producing and controlling the forces necessary for gripping branches or pushing off during gait.

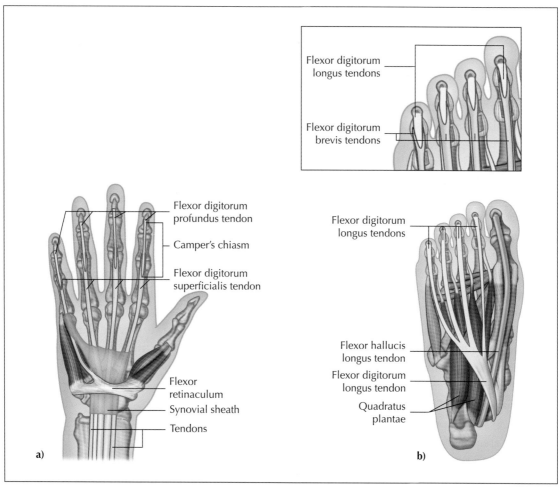

Figure 7.26. The tendons of the long finger (a) and toe (b) flexors pass through a tunnel provided by the shorter, deeper flexor tendons. This arrangement allows the bulkier and longer fibers to be positioned in the forearm and leg, which reduces the weight of the distal limbs and provides controlled movement through a longer range.

Each phalanx in the fingers and toes must move a little more than its more-proximal neighbor. Try flexing your fingers into a fist—the distal phalanges will always curl inward further than the proximal.[8] Control of the movement through that range requires longer muscle fibers, something that is difficult to host on the inherently short hand or foot.

The solution is to outsource the range of motion to the forearm and the leg with the long flexors and extensors that pass through the tendons of the shorter, deeper muscles to reach the distal phalanges (figure 7.26). Locating the muscles closer to the trunk allows them to build more bulk without increasing

---

[8]Unless you have had some form of injury, of course.

the weight of the hands and feet, which would increase the cost of movement, especially when running. This also allows for longer fiber lengths. If the muscles were limited to the length of the hands and feet, their fiber length and therefore their movement range would be significantly less, making it especially important for the finger and toe flexor muscles to originate on the forearm and leg, as they require both range and strength.

Summary

During the course of evolution, we developed many tools to help increase our range of movement through contralateral strategies. One of our greatest movement breakthroughs was developing to ability to connect and coordinate the rhythms between upper and opposite lower limb movement through the abdominal area. Our longer waist not only allows us to stand upright but also helps us use strain created through one limb to help pretension and support movement in the other limbs.

In earlier chapters, we have explored how tissue strain increases force and velocity outputs for the system (page 61) and how long-chain movements help increase leverage (page 45). Some of those connections are sagittal, such as the case of the softball pitcher (pages 42 and 67), and in this chapter we explored the benefit of contralateral movements and their connections, facilitated by the alternating oblique layers of abdominal muscles.

We saw both soft- and hard-tissue dynamics with the hand positioning of the footballers during the sprint decelerations, and neither dynamic is primary—they both occur simultaneously. Control of high-force long-chain movement can be enhanced through both soft-tissue strategies, such as the proposed continuities, and the coupling of bone movement.

The ability to see bone coupling during complex long-chain movement requires a separation of the language of bones and the language of joints. Although it may seem like pedantry at first, using the correct vocabulary allows your eyes to track exactly what is happening and where. In the next chapter we will take this a step further by clarifying the many ways we create movement through our joints.

Reflection Questions

1. How would you recognize a rotational muscle from its muscle fibers?
2. How do the upper and lower limbs relate to myofascial layers?
3. What is the significance of naming a bone or naming a joint when describing movement? Why is the language important?
4. What is the difference between describing joint movement in the limbs compared with movement of the spine?
5. Why might opposite hand and arm position be important for someone with "weak glutes"?

Notes

Layered anatomy and the effects of moving the limbs are woefully underexplored in the literature, as is the arrangement of complementary muscles that surround complex joints such as the hip and especially the shoulder. The shoulder girdle has a fascinating arrangement that makes total sense when it is pointed out that the superficial muscles (pectoralis major, latissimus dorsi, and trapezius) all cross each shoulder-girdle joint and connect to the other "limbs" for extra stability (pectorals connect to the opposite shoulder, latissimus to the lower limbs, and trapezius to the head). The next layer then has two sections—one that connects the scapula to the trunk (rhomboids, levator scapula, and serratus anterior), and one that connects the scapula to the humerus (the rotator cuff muscles). These layers surround the shoulder complex from each angle to provide range of movement and stability from every direction.

The stepping around exercises used in this chapter (e.g., figure 7.15) bring us back to the discussion on the foot and ankle complex. The talar joint allows flexion/ extension, and the subtalar joint allows inversion and eversion, but neither of them allows much rotation. The rotation created by stepping around is therefore coupled into the rest of the foot, which pronates or supinates depending on the direction of the rotation. Knowing the relationship between direction and strategy used for the movement therefore lets us predict the response of the foot and ankle.

For example, we could step the right foot to 4 o'clock and bend the left knee forward—a sagittal strategy and dorsiflexion reaction for the left ankle.

Or, we could step the right foot outward and back a little—a mostly frontal plane strategy that would invert the left subtalar joint.

Or, we could step the right foot around to 4 o'clock—a transverse plane strategy that would cause the left foot to pronate.

I suggest you try each of these to feel the difference. If you are not familiar with the functional anatomy of the foot and ankle, I would recommend my *Understanding the Human Foot* (Lotus, 2021).

Real and Relative Motion

8

How dreadful ... to be caught up in a game and have no idea of the rules.
—**Caroline Stevermer**, **Patricia C. Wrede**, *Sorcery and Cecelia*

Introduction

Much of the confusion in anatomy is simply about misunderstood, unexplained, or ill-defined terminology. As we have seen throughout this book, there are also conventions that are rarely disclosed or discussed, and life becomes much simpler once we appreciate the intended use of anatomical terminology. This, our last chapter together, will put the last few pieces of the puzzle into place for you so that you can read the whole book again with that promised new vision.

Yes, you read that correctly. I really recommend that you read the text again, because you will have even more vocabulary by the time you finish this chapter, vocabulary that provides clarity, facilitates

deeper understanding, and gifts the clearer vision promised at the beginning of this journey.

This chapter is possibly the most important of the book. Each chapter has introduced vocabulary and concepts to help us understand and appreciate the implications of movement direction, its drivers, and the associated forces. In the introductory chapters we saw that muscle can act concentrically, eccentrically, or isometrically, depending on the body's needs or its learned reactions, and how muscle actions have consequences beyond their anatomical borders. Muscle and fascial tissues are interweaved to produce structures that can adapt to the various movement needs, and the weaknesses of one tissue type are countered by the strengths of the other.

Fascia cannot contract quickly or with much force—that role is fulfilled by muscle fiber. But muscle fibers are structurally weak and cannot transfer force without breaking—therefore, they are reinforced by fascial tissues that allow some compliance. The compliance—or elasticity—not only protects the delicate muscle cells during movement but also enhances force output by adding more velocity during countermovement, stretch-shortening cycle, actions.

We have explored how movement travels through the body in quite predictable patterns in each plane, and now we get to practice the vocabulary and see the implications of movement variables. There are other forms of analysis and other vocabularies out there that add depth to the description of movement, especially in the world of dance—such as the work of Irmgard Bartenieff and Rudolf Laban, who separated out the mechanics and the *quality* of movement. Many movement disciplines need to describe the *experience* of movement, and there are evocative words to instill impressions, qualities, and characteristics of movement—all of which add important color to how a movement can be made.

Our aim here is to find the words that allow us to describe the reality of movement and link human movement to its anatomy. We have now introduced all the information and vocabulary you need to start to see anatomy in motion, and from that platform one can add further color regarding quality of movement, if desired. Our aim has been to build the skill to know the differences between "abducted" and "abducting" (e.g., in chapter 1), recognize variables that can influence movement through the body (chapter 2), understand the difference between stress and strain (chapter 3), become fluent with the cardinal directions, movement planes, and coupled motions (chapter 4), and the use of drivers and directions (chapter 5). To explore real-life

movement, we need to know the difference between range of motion, range of movement, and top-down/bottom-up directed movement (chapter 6), and the conventions of osteo- and arthrokinematics (chapter 7). Now, in this chapter we can pull them all together to see the mechanics of how our anatomy creates and responds to movement.

At first sight, the explanations and figures can seem a little confusing and the words may get in the way of seeing the importance of the concept. Take your time exploring each joint in turn, perform some of the movements to get the sense of what is happening, and remember that you might not do them in the same way someone else would. Keep in mind the intention of the movement and the target tissues. However, first we have to revisit some vocabulary.

Describing Bones and Joints

As Cuvier could correctly describe a whole animal by the contemplation of a single bone, so the observer who has thoroughly understood one link in a series of incidents should be able to accurately state all the other ones, both before and after.

— **Sir Arthur Conan Doyle**, *The Adventures of Sherlock Holmes*

Through clarity of thought and language, you too can have the deductive powers of Conan Doyle's famous detective, Sherlock Holmes. It is just a matter of piecing together the clues hidden in every movement to build the complete picture. The less famous George Cuvier (1769–1832), to whom Conan Doyle is referring here, was a pioneer of comparative anatomy with highly developed skills of interpretation of animal locomotion, which he could extrapolate from individual bones and their shapes.

Although we will not be looking at different species nor general locomotor patterns, you now have the skills to predict and describe most movement through the human body as it happens. To further build that skill, the previous chapter introduced osteo- and arthrokinematics in the transverse plane and emphasized the need for clarity on whether we were describing the movement of a bone or a joint. Differentiating between bone movement and joint movement is an essential step toward *seeing* anatomy in movement, and we can assist that process through precision of language— by accurately naming a bone or naming a joint and then describing its movement.

One of the issues for transverse plane movement is that we use the same term for both bone and joint movement—*rotation*. Sagittal and frontal plane motions reduce the potential for confusion because they both have technical terms for joint movement that do not translate to the bones. Flexion, extension, abduction, and adduction are all specific to the relationship at joints (figure 8.1). To *flex* or *extend* a bone would suggest the bone is bending or expanding, which would be changes in shape rather than position.[1] To *abduct* or *adduct* an individual bone would require its dislocation from all joints to allow it to move away from or closer to the midline.

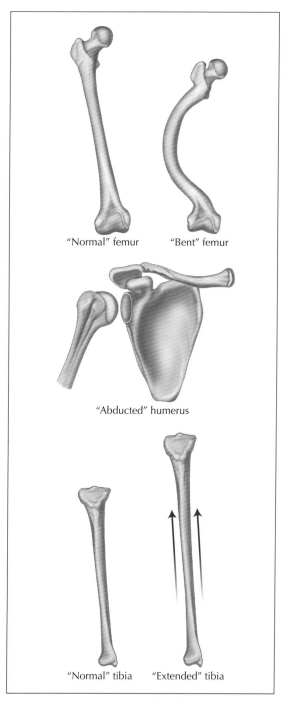

"Normal" femur   "Bent" femur

"Abducted" humerus

"Normal" tibia   "Extended" tibia

Figure 8.1. Terminology used for joint movements in the sagittal (flexion and extension) and frontal (abduction and adduction) planes is not generally used to describe movement of individual bones.

---

[1] Changes in bone shape can happen and are worthy of their own book.

There is a dissonance in sentences like: "Her femur is flexed," "His humerus is abducted," or "Their scapula is extended." Using joint movement descriptors for individual bones paints slightly disturbing images in a way that "rotation" does not—rotation works for both bone movement and joint relationship. Therefore, we will use slightly different terminology to describe sagittal and frontal plane movement of individual bones. Don't panic, it's simple.

Only two words are used to describe overall movement of the pelvis—it can either *tilt* or *rotate*. The pelvis rotates left and right (transverse plane), it tilts anteriorly and posteriorly (sagittal plane), and it tilts left and right (frontal plane), and we all know what is meant by those terms. As we already use *tilt* to describe the movement of a single structure (made up of a few bones, I know), why not apply the same convention to every other bone?

As single structures, the pelvis, thorax, and the head all tilt left and right. But paired structures, such as the humerus, femur, or tibia, will tilt medially and laterally. This change in language might seem a little strange at first, but have a look at figure 8.2 to explore the precision that can be gained from this simple change.

The scapula is another area where language is a little confused—some medical traditions use *upward* and *downward rotation* to describe what I call *medial* and *lateral tilting*. My objection to the use of upward and downward rotation is that, unless you already know the convention, it is not immediately obvious which plane of motion is being referred to.

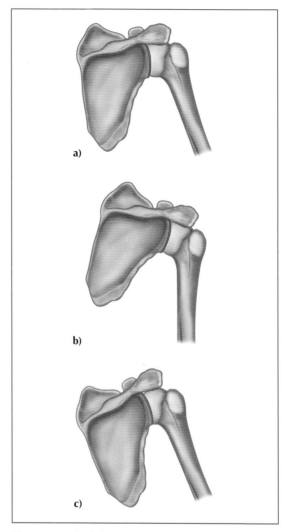

Figure 8.2. The joint arrangement in both (a) and (b) can be described as an abduction of the glenohumeral joint, but the ways in which they came about are quite different. Abduction of the glenohumeral joint happens when the angle between the scapula and humerus increases. Joint abduction can happen if the top of the humerus tilts toward the scapula (a), or the scapula tilts toward the humerus (b). It is rare during normal movement for only one bone to move and both bones could move the same amount in the same direction and no relative movement happens at the glenohumeral joint (c).

"Upward rotation" could be an equally valid descriptor for the front of the scapula to face upward (figure 8.3), a sagittal plane motion rather than a frontal plane one.

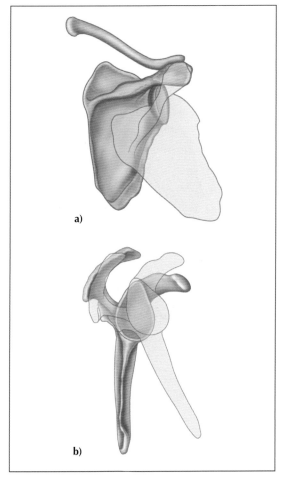

Figure 8.3. Upward and downward rotation are commonly used descriptors for movement of the scapula (a). However, those terms could be misinterpreted as posterior and anterior tilt of the scapula (b), as the front of the scapula is "rotated" upward or downward. Using "tilt" to describe changes in the vertical orientation allows us to describe the four positions shown in (a) and (b) as laterally, medially, posteriorly, and anteriorly tilted, which is much more consistent and easily interpreted.

One could argue that the language you choose does not really matter provided it is consistent and precise, but language must facilitate communication between professionals. Therefore, I choose to use "tilt" to describe deviations in the sagittal and frontal planes because it matches our common everyday usage (things tilt forward and back, left and right), and it adapts easily to the anatomical conventions of describing single structures with left and right, paired structures with medial and lateral.

Describing the tilt of bones also helps me explain and explore the five ways we change the relationship at joints in the sagittal and frontal planes, and reserve the terms *abduction, adduction, flexion,* and *extension* for joint relationships.

Five Ways to Create Motion at Joints

When I was first taught the language and vision of relative joint motion during my training with the Gray Institute, I got a little angry and a little depressed that it had taken me so long to find this out. At first sight the language and the directions seemed confusing, but gradually I saw there is a beautiful, clear, and very useful logic to how the system is laid out.

Since learning from Gray and Tiberio, I have seen a couple of other attempts to create methods to describe joint motion, but none of them has the same level of clarity and consistency. If you have not come across osteo- and arthrokinematics before, the language can seem contrived, but the reality is that it slots in perfectly because it is an extension of standard anatomical conventions. This is not new language, but few people know how to use it accurately and precisely.

Although the title of this section promises five movements, there are seven possibilities of movement at joints:

1. The distal bone moves, and the proximal bone remains in place (figure 8.2a).
2. The distal bone stays in place, and the proximal bone moves (figure 8.2b).
3. Both bones move in one direction, but the distal moves further.
4. Both bones move in the other direction, but the proximal bone moves further.
5. Both bones move in opposite directions.
6. No movement occurs: neither bone moves, so nothing happens at the level of the joint.
7. Both bones move in the same direction and at the same speed (figure 8.2c). The result is that no changes in length occur in the tissues that cross the joint, but the soft tissues will experience some degree of change in tone to stabilize the relationship between the bones. So, even though no relative motion occurs, the tissue may alter its degree of strain.

No relative motion occurs in 6 and 7, but there is an important difference between them. In the last example, if movement is occurring through the body and a joint is deliberately stabilized, the direction in which the force approaches the joint will affect which tissues work more to stabilize. For example, a ballerina must be able to pirouette turning toward and away from the standing leg (figure 8.4), and, although each muscle will be engaged, the clockwise or anticlockwise spin

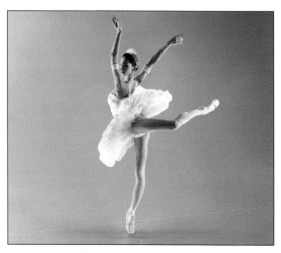

Figure 8.4. As the pelvis and thorax remain relatively neutral to each other during a pirouette, the direction of spin will determine which line of obliques works a little harder to maintain the relationship. Visualize the implications of whether the spin is initiated by the arms (top-down) or from a push from the nonsupporting leg (bottom-up).[3] How does the direction of movement impulse change the line of strain? What happens if the pelvis receives the impulse before the rib cage or vice versa?

will require different degrees of tone from opposite sides of the joints.[2]

What Is All the Fuss About?

When a man's knowledge is not in order, the more of it he has the greater will be his confusion.

—Herbert Spencer,
The Study of Sociology

---

[2] The terminology in ballet is *en dehors* and *en dedans*; turning away from and toward, respectively.
[3] For those of you who know ballet, this is just intended as a thought exercise and not as an instruction on how to perform a pirouette, and I apologize for abusing your beautiful art form.

Confusing bone movement with joint reaction is probably one of the most common types of confusion I see among therapists. I had to practice being deliberate with my descriptors when teaching classes to differentiate between naming bones and naming joints. As mentioned above, for the first 20 years of my practice, I did not even know the significance of the difference between them—my knowledge was not in order. However, once I practiced the vocabulary, it was as though blinkers had been removed, and I could see and describe movement with confidence and accuracy.

Knowing the five ways to create a specific motion at any joint also helped me be more creative when working with clients. If there was a problem with certain muscles but I wanted to create motion at their associated joint, I could use novel strategies to bypass dysfunctional or challenged tissues. By understanding how the joints react we can direct movement with or without active concentric contraction of the agonists, we can stimulate the antagonists, use momentum from other body parts, or any combination of strategies to bring movement to a target joint or tissue.

The examples below are deliberately chosen to highlight the many ways we can "lengthen" the shoulder adductors, the hip extensors, and the lateral rotators of the hip. Each movement can create the same line of strain through the three areas, but the strategy to achieve that strain is very different in each case.

Try the movements if you can, play with them, but don't allow yourself to become frustrated if they don't make sense at first.

Note:
- Movement has already taken place in most of this series of images.
- Bones that have moved are highlighted with a red arrow.
- If a bone does not move it is shown in green.
- The direction of tilt is indicated by the top of the arrow.
- When two bones have moved, the bone that moves further is indicated by the thicker arrow.
- The first example in each of the three series of demonstrations of relative motion shows us the textbook normal—the distal bone moves away from a static proximal bone. They therefore demonstrate the concentric contraction of the muscle of the associated group.

The demonstrations that follow will highlight many of the other forces that cooperate to produce similar end positions but are driven by a range of other muscles and forces. The first movement for each example is the textbook action—the distal bone moves away from the proximal using a concentric muscle contraction. The other methods of producing the joint relationship will recruit a variety of other strategies, some of which might not even require active engagement of the muscles normally associated with the action.

Abduct the Glenohumeral Joint

Abduction of the glenohumeral joint means that the angle between the humerus and the scapula increases and we have five ways this can happen:

Medially tilting the humerus (figure 8.5) is the usual way we would think about creating abduction at the glenohumeral joint.

Laterally tilting the scapula (figure 8.6) is an ideal example of how we could create joint motion indirectly by using other body parts that cause the proximal bone to move. As the left arm comes up and across overhead, it causes the rib cage, and therefore the right scapula, to tilt to the right (laterally).

The right glenohumeral joint abducts because the scapula tilts relative to the humerus.

If you are unsure about the relationship, tilt the page until the red arrow on the scale is horizontal. You will then see that the two arrows match those in the previous illustration (although the colors are swapped).

In this case, the right glenohumeral joint abducts because of the movement of the left arm and subsequent tilt of the rib cage.

In theory, the muscles around the right shoulder joint could be relaxed and uninvolved in the movement—the joint abduction results from momentum created through the left upper limb.

Most everyday movements and many exercises will cause both bones to move (figure 8.7). In this case, both the scapula and the humerus are tilting medially—in the same direction—as the right arm swings outward and overhead and the scapula tilts along with the rib cage. As the humerus moves further than the scapula, the glenohumeral joint abducts.

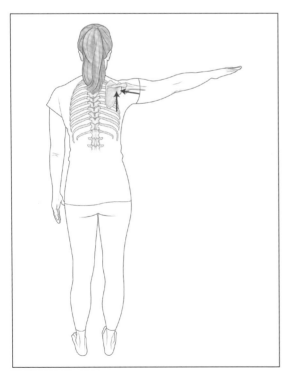

Figure 8.5. Medially tilt the humerus.

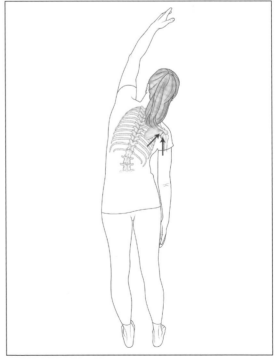

Figure 8.6. Laterally tilt the scapula.

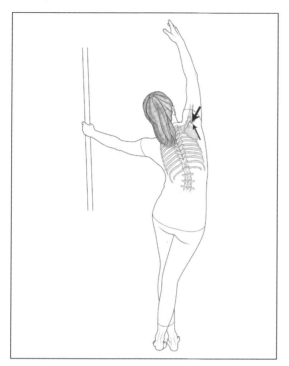

Figure 8.7. Medially tilt both the humerus and the scapula, but tilt the humerus more.

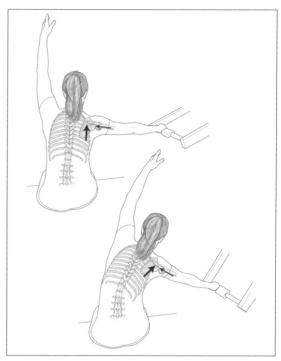

Figure 8.8. Laterally tilt both bones, but the scapula tilts further.

Almost every medial tilt of the humerus caused by the deltoid and other glenohumeral abductors will eventually draw the scapula into a medial tilt. According to the textbooks, the first 60 degrees (approximately) of glenohumeral abduction is generally achieved through movement of the humerus (as in figure 8.5). Beyond 60 degrees, the scapula tilts medially to allow the glenoid fossa to travel along with the head of the humerus and maintain joint integrity. But this is an anatomy story, and most people do not isolate the humerus from the scapula through the early stages of the movement—the scapula and humerus cooperate from the beginning of most normal actions.

Also, as with most joint movements, glenohumeral abduction does not occur on a single plane—the humerus will laterally rotate as it abducts to allow the movement.

I recommend investigating the literature dealing with scapulohumeral rhythm for further information, but also as an exercise to reveal the inconsistencies in the use of descriptors for bone and joint movement.

When starting a movement from an abducted position, the humerus can laterally tilt (which would normally create an **ad**duction of the glenohumeral joint), but the scapula can also tilt laterally and could tilt further than the humerus (figure 8.8).

Figure 8.7 shows how the right scapula reacts to the movement driven by the left arm as it reaches over and across the head.

As the right arm is pressing down on the bar, the glenohumeral **ad**ductors are engaged eccentrically to control the **ab**duction.

As the trunk tilts to the right to follow the left arm, the right scapula will tilt laterally. The right tilt of the trunk causes the right shoulder area to drop toward the floor, and, as the hand is fixed on the pole, the movement of the torso causes the right humerus to tilt medially.

Fixing the right hand, as in this case, and driving movement from the opposite shoulder complex is an excellent strategy for mobilizing the right shoulder area without involving much contraction of the muscles surrounding it.

Similar strategies can be employed by using the lower limbs to mobilize the upper limbs or vice versa.

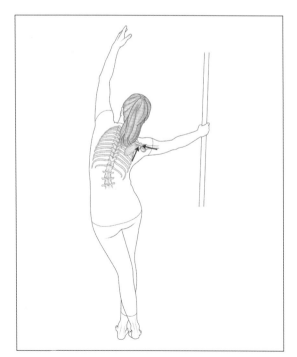

Figure 8.9. Laterally tilt the scapula and medially tilt the humerus.

Flex the Hip Joint

Flexion of the hip means that the angle at the front of the hip joint decreases. We have five ways in which that can happen:

Staying true to the open-chain anatomy texts, a simple leg lift will flex the hip by tilting the femur posteriorly (figure 8.10). Although one could argue over the ability to totally isolate the femur from the pelvis, for this example we will assume the left innominate bone did not move.

An anterior tilt of the pelvis (figure 8.11) creates the same relationship at the hip joint as a posterior tilt of the femur—I hope that is obvious by now. However, the muscle actions and the potential ranges of motion can be very different.

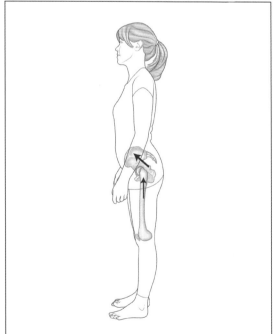

Figure 8.10. Posteriorly tilt the femur.

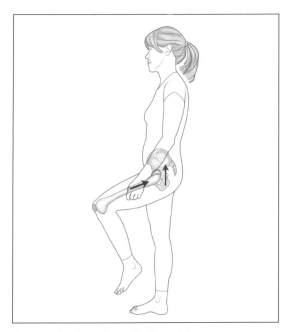

Figure 8.11. Anteriorly tilt the pelvis.

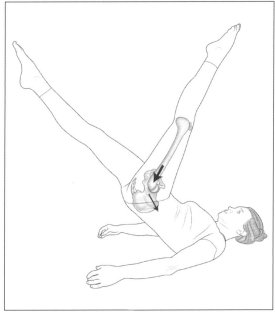

Figure 8.12. Posteriorly tilt both pelvis and femur, but tilt the femur more.

Experience the two movements to feel the difference. How far can you lift your leg (figure 8.9), compared with how far you can tilt your pelvis forward (figure 8.10)?

Although they are the same movement at the hip joint, the movement of the pelvis has more implications for the lumbar spine position.

> How did your strategies change between the two movements?
> Which muscles were used more or less in each movement?
> How many different strategies can you use to create both movements?

As hinted at in the first example, most open-chain movements will involve movement of more than one bone. It is a fact of our connectedness that neighboring bones are likely to follow along when one moves. Preventing them from doing so

can be taught as part of a discipline to enhance movement aesthetics for dance or performance, or to enhance motor control and awareness.

Although one cue for this Pilates-based exercise might be to "stabilize" the pelvis, the left innominate is likely to follow the posterior tilt of the femur (figure 8.12). Although the left innominate is posteriorly tilting, the femur tilts further, creating flexion at the hip joint.

The starting position for the exercise—with both feet on the bar—creates an interesting dynamic in that the movement toward hip flexion is initiated by a concentric contraction of the hip flexors until the left lower limb passes vertical. The change in relationship with gravity then causes the work to switch across to the hip extensors, which will control the movement through eccentric contraction.

There are many ways of entering the Downward Dog Pose and figures 8.13 and 8.14 show two of them.

In figure 8.13, the forward fold at the hip causes the pelvis to tilt anteriorly. The pelvis then follows the hands as they walk forward, the femurs are also drawn anteriorly, but the pelvis has still tilted further than the femurs, and the hips stay in flexion.

You might notice that the hip is more flexed by the forward bend (figure 8.13a) than in the final position (figure 8.13c). The deeper flexion is reduced as the hands walk forward, causing the hips to extend but without going into extension (review the "Vocabulary Builder" in chapter 1 if that is unclear).

Note: The eagle-eyed among you will also notice that the femur initially tilts posteriorly as the pelvis tilts forward, which connects us to the hip-flexion final sequence.

Movement analysis is often performed according to the final position rather than in context of how the body got there. Knowing the starting position is crucial to an understanding of what might have happened through the system as it moved.

Most people will recognize the yoga asana of Downward Dog and the two pictures of the final position (figures 8.13 and 8.14) are

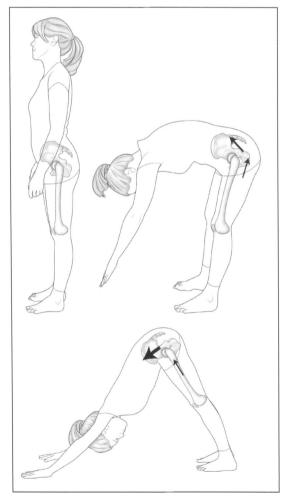

Figure 8.13. Anteriorly tilt both bones but the pelvis more.

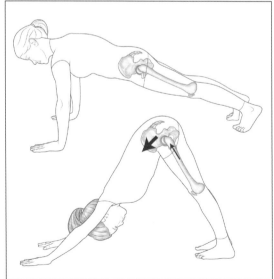

Figure 8.14. Anteriorly tilt the pelvis and posteriorly tilt the femur.

almost identical, but the primary muscles used to get there are quite different.

Because a plank was used as the starting position in figure 8.14, rather than a standing forward bend (as in figure 8.13), the femurs move into a posterior tilt and the pelvis tilts anteriorly—the combination of figures 8.10 and 8.11 above.

Although the entry to the pose might be different, the direction of the line of strain along the back will remain the same. However, the entry strategy might change where the strain is focused. I recommend experimenting with yourself and with clients to compare individual responses.

Medially Rotate the Hip

Starting off with the easy and familiar open-chain reaction, a medial rotation of the right hip can be created by medially rotating the right femur (figure 8.15) …

… or we could turn the pelvis to the right (figure 8.16).

Stepping the left foot around to the right will cause the pelvis to turn to the right as well, and medial rotation will take place at the right hip.

Once again, we could have the discussion over movement isolation—it is likely that the right femur will laterally rotate owing to the momentum from the pelvis, but the pelvis will rotate further, and the hip will still be medially rotated.

The lift and reach of the right leg cause the femur to rotate medially and, eventually, the pelvis will follow by rotating to the left (the same direction as the femur; figure 8.17). As the movement started from below, from the leg and foot, it is the distal bones that are rotating further than the proximal bones to create medial rotation at the right hip joint.

This is the same exercise as figure 8.17 but is led by the left leg rather than the right. However, it still causes the right hip to go into medial rotation, as the pelvis reacts to the movement of the left leg by lifting slightly on the left and rotating toward the right femur. The right femur will follow the pelvis to the right but, because the pelvis is following the larger movement of the left leg, the pelvis will rotate further than the femur.

The movements in figures 8.17 and 8.18 are perfect examples of the difference between bottom-up- (figure 8.17) and top-down-directed (figure 8.18) movement.

In figure 8.17 the right femur is directing the movement upward to the right hip joint (bottom-up). In figure 8.18, it is the pelvis directing the movement of the right femur (top-down).

The top-down example shown here can be a little confusing as the left foot is driving the movement upward to the left hip and into the pelvis, but the right hip is responding to the movement of the pelvis (top-down).

A posterior lunge with internal rotation of the right foot causes the pelvis to rotate to the right. As with the previous three examples

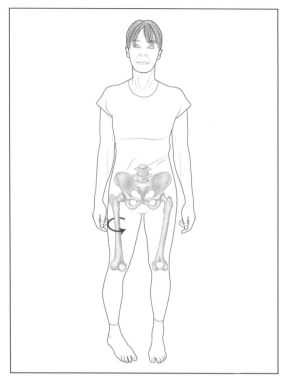

Figure 8.15. The femur rotates medially.

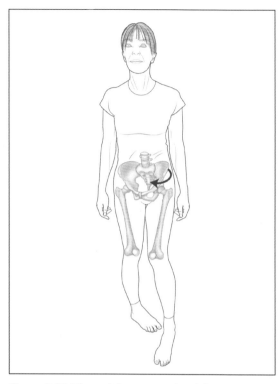

Figure 8.16. The pelvis turns to the right.

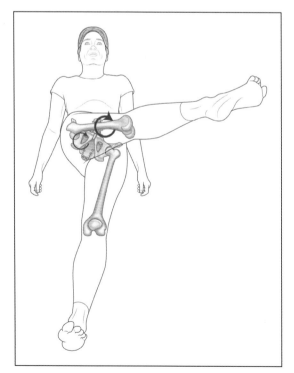

Figure 8.17. Both bones medially rotate.

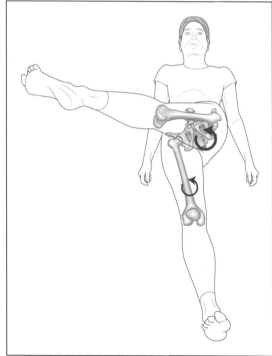

Figure 8.18. Both bones laterally rotate.

of relative motions, this final example where the bones move in opposite directions is a composite of the first two motions—a medial rotation of the femur and a right rotation of the pelvis (figure 8.19).

However, compare the strategies for causing the pelvis to turn—in (figure 8.16) the left foot stepped around, while in this example the same-side leg stepped back.

This example can bring us back to the discussion about the use of sagittal, frontal, and transverse planes of motion. Because of the offset between the central line of the torso and the off-center attachment of the limbs, the predominantly sagittal plane motion of one

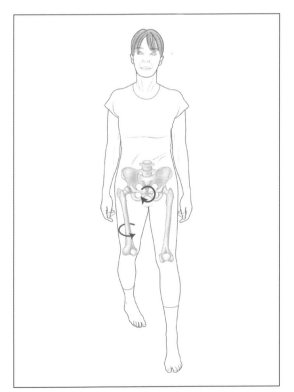

Figure 8.19. Both bones move in opposite directions.

limb causes the trunk to rotate to let it reach forward or back.

Now compare the reaction of the pelvis as the left leg steps forward in (figure 8.15) with the posterior step in (figure 8.16)—the opposite limbs rotate the pelvis in the same direction.

Five Strategies to Affect the Same Tissues

Taking time to work through the examples above, to answer the reflection questions, and to create your own "five ways to …" (insert an action and a joint of your choice) exercises will be time well spent. Not only will it expand your movement repertoire by opening new possibilities for mobilizing, strengthening, and stretching any area, but it also provides a full tensegrity understanding of how the body interacts.

For example, take any of the movements above and consider how the joint motion was created. There are many strategies that could be followed but these will cover most of them:

1. **Active concentric contraction**—drawing the distal bone toward the proximal
2. **Active concentric contraction**—drawing the proximal bone toward the distal
3. Very little, if any, contraction if a motion is created through **gravity**, although this often needs to be controlled by an eccentric muscle contraction
4. **Momentum** created after a countermovement lengthened the tissues on the opposite side of the joint
5. **Distal muscle action** creating a motion that causes a joint to react

6. A combination of factors—**concentric contraction**, gravity, **momentum**, and **distal drivers**.

Can you match the movements above to each of the possible reactions?

Joining the Dots and Getting Creative

Quotes are like prompts. A way of searching, connecting the dots.
—**Masha Tupitsyn, interview on** *Culture.org*

Congratulations—you now have all the tools you need to see, understand, and even direct movement.

The above examples have built on the skills we have used through the book—drivers, directions, planes, and tissue reactions. Think about the relationship between the desired joint movements and the directions in which we used other drivers to create the reaction.

Our first example, glenohumeral abduction, uses frontal plane motions of a variety of drivers to cause a frontal plane action. The same is true for the next two examples—hip flexion in the sagittal plane and hip rotation in the transverse plane. If you want to create a joint action in one of the major planes, simply request movement from another body part in the same plane. Of course, there will be the occasional plane changes, as we saw with the unilateral limb movement in the sagittal plane, which caused the body to rotate (e.g., figure 8.19).

When movement is cued gently and with attention to the safety and comfort of the client, the process can take on a trial-and-error approach, as you both explore the various reactions. The therapist keeps a watchful eye on the client to look for smooth and appropriate dispersal of strain through their body as they perform any action. Think of the overall range of movement and consider the contribution from each tissue—does each tissue contribute accordingly? Is there a pleasant rhythm through each section of the body? Or is there an area or two that draw your eye?

It does not matter whether you first notice too much or too little movement in an area. Sometimes a rib or a knee, for example, will stand out because it is moving more than we expected—other times we might notice the quiet area. What is important is that we take the next step and find the reason—if something is moving too much, there must be an area that is contributing less, and vice versa.

Be sure to identify each section through the chain and then consider how you could adapt the exercise to encourage more movement into the area that needs it. There is no repertoire for this, there are just the principles that we have explored. If you want a repertoire there are many, many books that cover the same old "stretches"—but you chose to learn about the principles of movement for a reason. You want to move above and beyond the simplified repetition of standard positions, and—remember—you wanted to learn to fish, and, like any skill, fishing takes practice.

As mentioned often, this book can also be taken at two levels—for movement ideas to help clients, and to help you *see* movement and anatomy more clearly. The vocabulary and the exercises are the principles that will allow you to do that.

We have busted many of the myths of anatomy-book-based anatomy. We have seen that not all movement is made up of concentric actions. We have clarified the language of anatomy and explored how myofascial tissues work to help long-chain movement. By looking at our common countermovement strategies we have seen how the human body adapts to improve its leverage for more powerful actions and what happens when the limbs and the head are moved. We have used the language of drivers— provided by the Gray Institute—to explore the implications of direction through the sagittal, frontal, and transverse planes.

Importantly, we have defined what is meant by each of the words we use. The planes of motion are not restricted to paper-thin lines but are tools to give us the power to predict the reactions through the body and how they correlate to the main joint actions of flexion/ extension, abduction/adduction, and rotation. Grasping that vocabulary is the beginning to a new vision of the full body in action—a powerful tool that, once seen, begins to transcend vocabulary so no words are needed, but learning the words provides the vital initial vision and understanding.

Although I claim absolutely no prowess in filling every sentence with an "overflow of meaning, and … many resonances," I will leave the final guidance to the great author Hilary Mantel (who sadly passed away as I came to the end of writing this text).

> *Some readers read a book as if it were an instruction manual, expecting to understand everything first time, but of course when you write, you put into every sentence an overflow of meaning, and you create in every sentence as many resonances and double meanings and ambiguities as you can possibly pack in there, so that people can read it again and get something new each time.*
> —**Hilary Mantel, interview for the *New Statesman***

I hope to see you next time around.